'This is a sensit   )le for all health
professionals carir.   , and their families.
Based on current research and the experience of skilled spiritual
care practitioners, this text comprises numerous practical examples
and strategies that will provide a solid methodology and a valuable
assessment guide for those wanting to add depth or another dimension
to the quality of their care.'

*— Dr Lindsay Carey, MAppSc, PhD, Research Fellow in Palliative
Care and Head of Public Health Major, School of Psychology and
Public Health, La Trobe University, Melbourne, Australia, and
Co-Editor,* Health and Social Care Chaplaincy, *UK*

'This is a recommended read and a much-needed resource for anyone
involved in caring for sick children and young people. For far too long
there has been a deficit in this specific field and dimension of practice.
The authors should be congratulated for providing an engaging and
informative text supporting the integration of spiritual care within
everyday practice all the while keeping the voice and needs of the sick
child and young person and their families at the centre of all interaction.'

*— Wilf McSherry, Professor in Dignity of Care for Older People,
Staffordshire University, The Shrewsbury and Telford Hospital
NHS Trust and Haraldsplass Deaconess University College*

'This book demonstrates how essential it is to have spiritual care
integrated in multi-professional practice to address this much neglected
dimension of holistic care. With 27 years in the field, I am certain
that a cancer diagnosis causes spiritual pain and suffering for children,
young people and their families. In the modern Western world, largely
distrustful or disconnected from religion, we have lost our spiritual
language. The authors offer us simple and effective tools to connect in
a spiritual way with those we care for. If you are at all uncertain read
page 149 first.'

*— Jeanette Hawkins RGN, RSCN, DPSN, MSc Advanced
Nursing Practice, Assistant Director, CLIC Sargent*

'Paul Nash, Kathryn Darby and Sally Nash offer a book borne of the intense and awe-filled experience of listening to children and young people who have dis-ease. This is the kind of book I wish had been available when I became a paediatric chaplain over 20 years ago – examples, potential activities and most of all the spiritual reflection that can only be done by people who have been at the hospital bedside. It is in the act of play that we become who we truly are, and these playful activities aim to facilitate wholeness by helping children and youth connect with their core identity and become their healthy – whole – selves.'

— Daniel H. Grossoehme, DMin, MS, BCC, Associate Professor of Pediatrics (Research) and Staff Chaplain III, Cincinnati Children's Hospital Medical Center, Cincinnati, Ohio, USA

'This handbook is a valuable and timely addition to the literature, given that, today, much attention is being given to the role of spirituality in holistic health care and wellbeing. The topics are relevant and have been carefully informed by current research and the extensive use of story both illuminates and inspires the work. The writing is accessible and the wide array of activities and strategies offered by the authors make this book particularly useful for parents and care workers alike.'

— Marian de Souza, Chair, International Association for Children's Spirituality

SPIRITUAL CARE
with Sick Children and Young People

SPIRITUAL CARE

with Sick Children and Young People

*A handbook for chaplains,
paediatric health professionals,
arts therapists and youth workers*

Paul Nash, Kathryn Darby and Sally Nash

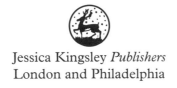

Jessica Kingsley *Publishers*
London and Philadelphia

Song on page 139 reproduced from Carson and WGRG (1998) by kind permission. Guatemalan traditional, translation © 1998 Christine Carson & WGRG, Iona Community, arrangement © 1998 WGRG, Iona Community, Glasgow G2 3DH, Scotland. wgrg@iona.org.uk; www.wgrg.co.uk.

First published in 2015
by Jessica Kingsley Publishers
73 Collier Street
London N1 9BE, UK
and
400 Market Street, Suite 400
Philadelphia, PA 19106, USA

www.jkp.com

Library of Congress Cataloging in Publication Data
Nash, Paul, 1959- , author.
Spiritual care with sick children and young people : a handbook for chaplains, paediatric health professionals, arts therapists, and youth workers / Paul Nash, Kathryn Darby, and Sally Nash.
p. ; cm.
Includes bibliographical references and index.
ISBN 978-1-84905-389-1 (alk. paper)
I. Darby, Kathryn, 1964- , author. II. Nash, Sally, 1957- , author. III. Title.
[DNLM: 1. Spiritual Therapies--methods. 2. Spirituality. 3. Adolescent. 4. Child. 5. Pastoral Care. 6. Young Adult. WB 885]
BT732.5
615.8'52--dc23
2015014877

British Library Cataloguing in Publication Data
A CIP catalogue record for this book is available from the British Library

ISBN 978 1 84905 389 1
eISBN 978 1 78450 063 4

Printed and bound in Great Britain

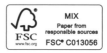

This book is dedicated to the children, young people,
families and staff who shared the journey
of exploring spiritual care with us.

Contents

Preface

This book has emerged out of the spiritual care practice of the Chaplaincy Team at Birmingham Children's Hospital NHS Foundation Trust (BCH) although it draws on a much wider network inside and outside of the hospital in providing inspiration, encouragement, advice, support and stories. Some of the team would say that engaging in spiritual care in this way has transformed their practice.

We are grateful to those who have contributed both practice examples and activities to this book; it makes it so much richer. Where we have permission to use actual names of children and young people we have done this, otherwise they are pseudonyms. We did not set out to write a book of resources, but we hope you find the stories that we tell of work with children, young people and families and the activities that we describe an encouragement to you in your own practice. While this is a book about work with sick children, many of the activities and examples will have a relevance beyond this setting.

We acknowledge that there is an overlap between what this book calls spiritual care and other disciplines where a different name may be used for a similar type of activity, such as psychosocial care. We want to celebrate this and see it as synergetic – not doing the same job, but mutually respecting each other's professions and working in multidisciplinary teams towards the wellbeing of the sick child or young person.

We work with children and young people aged 0–18 and when we specifically use the term 'child' we mean someone under 11; a 'young person' is 11–18. 'Children and young people' includes all young people up to age 18. We use the term 'sick' inclusively to encompass injury, disability, life-limiting conditions and illness, incorporating both physical and mental health issues. Where applicable we give specific contexts in our practice examples. 'Spiritual care practitioner' is used to mean a member of staff from any discipline who is engaging in spiritual care with a child or young person. We note the specific discipline where appropriate.

We hope this book offers readers the opportunity to gain a deeper understanding of the potential spiritual issues and needs faced by sick children and young people and to feel better equipped and confident in engaging in spiritual care in an intentional way. We hope too that we communicate how much we gain from encounters with unique, beautiful and courageous children, young people and their families; we are so often deeply moved by the insights we glimpse into their worlds.

This book is a joint endeavour by the three authors. While the chapters were divided between us and we each took a lead on particular ones, the book is a collaborative project and we share ownership of what we have written.

If you are interested in training or visiting BCH to experience the spiritual care we offer please contact the Centre for Paediatric Spiritual Care on cpscbch@gmail.com.

All proceeds from this book will be used for spiritual care work at Birmingham Children's Hospital.

Chapter 1

Introduction to Spiritual Care

PRACTICE EXAMPLE 1.1: RIA'S BOX

Liz visited 11-year-old Ria on a neurological ward. Ria has spent all her life in and out of hospital for surgery and treatment. She has some difficulty with fine motor skills and sometimes uses a wheelchair. Ria's experience has given her a wisdom and maturity about life that was reflected in the activity of decorating a small oval box. Though somewhat low spirited when Liz arrived, she swiftly perked up and chatted freely as materials were unpacked and activity began. The creative activity became a catalyst for expressing her thoughts and Ria described her frequent visits to the hospital, and some of the pressures her family had been experiencing. Liz produced a bag with a few items in for Ria to choose from. They talked about what Ria might keep in her box, with the suggestion that Ria might write her worries on one of the little cards in the bag and put them in the box. Ria then chose a pearl and gold-wire heart, saying, 'It sparkles and makes me feel happy.' Ria then chose a clear glass pebble saying it made her think of the sea. Liz and Ria spoke of how love is like the waves of the sea that never stop rolling in and how that can represent taking those worries and enfolding them in love and carrying them away. Ria held the glass pebble and said, 'I'm not really a religious person but I feel as if this is speaking to me.' There was a clear sense of exploring spirituality and transcendence. Liz comments, 'By creating a safe space and by listening there is a depth of connection that God's presence brings as I care for patients and families – creating that safe space is vital.'

Uninterrupted time, suggests Liz, 'is a gift and this facilitated Ria's freedom to open up and talk freely.' As the importance of spiritual care is recognised as part of a multidisciplinary approach to care, spiritual care practitioners can safeguard such spaces, scheduling in time alongside other professionals. Liz observed that Ria had a profound awareness of matters of death, learning through adversity, facing difficulty, recognising her own vulnerability, and finding glimmers of light and hope in the midst of long-term challenge. At the end of the session, there was a shared sense of spirits lifted as Ria rested the glass pebble on the tissue paper lining her small box.

Liz Bryson, spiritual care volunteer

One of the main insights we have learnt from our work is that *spiritual care is much easier to explore than explain*, which is why we have started this book with one of many stories or practice examples. However, we have tried to articulate what it is that we do and how we explain spiritual care in relation to work with sick children, young people and their families. It is a working, organic definition; what some may call a phenomenological definition. There are elements within it that are integral to any healthcare, such as dignity and respect, but we have included such facets here to reinforce their importance.

Every child and young person who comes into our care at Birmingham Children's Hospital is a spiritual as well as physical being who has *unique features, interests, skills and hopes and a unique personality*. Each one should be treated with *dignity, respect and compassion*.

Children and young people will value *being listened to, taken seriously* and *feeling connected* to others.

They benefit from *being included* in social groups and activities when they wish, particularly if they feel a *sense of loss, boredom or isolation*, and may appreciate being given the opportunity to make a *contribution to others* and to society.

Staff can contribute to a child's or young person's developing sense of their *own unique value by empowerment*, and by *developing and respecting their autonomy*.

We cannot underestimate the importance of *building rapport and trust*, and taking an interest in the *unique person* receiving treatment. They may wish to draw upon some recognised *religious beliefs or worldview*, or a mixture of several, to draw comfort and direction from, and staff will be able to support this.

Enhanced privacy and the *opportunity for social interaction with peers* is highly valued by young people.

Providing a positive space is an important part of providing spiritual care.

Helping children and young people find a 'new normal' may take a number of turns and involve setbacks, and readapting along the way. We propose that all this may be done within the wider context of the child's family too.

A definitive cure is sometimes elusive; consequently, young people may be *wrestling with important questions* about such things as suffering, identity, sexuality, meaning, purpose, life and death. Spiritual care involves helping children and young people by using *interpretive spiritual encounters* to discuss the difficult and complex aspects of the journey, as well as the more positive points of *meaning and connection* to be found along the way. Such discussions may help mitigate spiritual pain and distress, which may be experienced as a consequence of being sick.

There is a range of approaches to, and understandings of, spiritual care and related concepts, such as spirituality and spiritual need, and in the remainder of this chapter we will explore some brief exemplars which give an idea of the breadth of current thought. The research on paediatric spiritual care is not extensive. As part of a wider systematic literature review Paul identified the following as significant: Bull and Gillies (2007); Bull (2013); Campbell (2006); Darby, Nash and Nash (2014a, 2014b); Erickson (2008); Feudtner, Haney and Dimmers (2003); Grossoehme (1996, 1999, 2008); Grossoehme, Cotton and Leonard (2007); Grossoehme, VanDyke and Seid (2008); Grossoehme, Szczesniak, McPhail and Seid (2013); Nash, Nash and Frith (2011); Nash, Darby and Nash (2013); Pridmore and Pridmore (2004). Some of the insights from this research, which have informed our own work, include:

- the importance of finding appropriate approaches to spiritual assessment (Grossoehme 2008)

- the way that children and young people often use a different vocabulary to express their spiritual experience, and the importance of understanding developmental stages (Grossoehme 1999)

- the large number of parents who have specific needs, which also need assessing (Feudtner *et al.* 2003)

- the reciprocal nature of relationships and potential for spiritual distress (Pridmore and Pridmore 2004)

- the importance of helping children and young people see that the body has spiritual significance (Grossoehme *et al.* 2008)

- the significance of dreams, aspirations, hope and connectedness in sickness (Erickson 2008)

- that spiritual needs may include religious beliefs, and it is the role of all healthcare professionals to try to identify and meet these needs (Bull and Gillies 2007)

- the importance of play in relating to sick children (Bull 2013)

- facilitating religious observance (Campbell 2006).

It is not possible within the scope of this book to offer a detailed understanding of the spirituality of children and young people but there are a range of texts which provide good summaries (e.g. Adams, Hyde and Woolley 2008; Hay and Nye 2006; Hyde 2008).

Spirituality

Spirituality is a contested concept with a plurality of definitions across disciplines and contexts. Within a healthcare context, the Association of American Medical Colleges provides a useful, succinct definition in relation to spiritual care, which arose out of a consensus conference including clinicians, chaplains and medical educators in 1999. It states that: 'spirituality is the aspect of humanity that refers to the way individuals seek and express meaning and purpose, and the way they experience their connectedness to the moment, to self, to others, to nature and to the significant or sacred' (Puchalski and Ferrell 2010, p.25). This is a generic definition, which could apply to children and young people or spiritual care practitioners regardless of worldview or faith.

Spiritual needs

Narayanasamy (2010) highlights Maslow's hierarchy of needs in his discussion of spiritual needs. The hierarchy of having basic needs met first (physiological; food and drink, sleep), followed by safety (feeling secure), social (belonging to a group, feeling loved), self-esteem (self-respect) and, finally, by self-actualisation (growth, personal development), can inform our understanding of spiritual needs and wellbeing. He challenges the idea of a hierarchy, where some needs can appear more important than others, but refers to it as a useful framework which relates to spiritual needs.

Narayanasamy (2010) suggests we express our spiritual needs in a variety of ways:

- the need for meaning and purpose

- the need for love and harmonious relationships

- the need for forgiveness

- the need for a source of hope and strength

- the need for trust

- the need for expression of personal beliefs and values

- the need for spiritual practices, expression of the concept of God or deity and creativity.

While these identified needs are in no way exhaustive, they are increasingly recognised within healthcare as part of holistic care and can be seen as significant in relation to the impact on physical health. One of the things we are particularly interested in researching further is the way that the normative spiritual needs of children and young people are affected by or added to because of their illness.

Nursing perspectives

In the UK, the Royal College of Nursing offers this definition in a publication on spirituality in nursing (drawing on the work of NHS Education for Scotland). Spiritual care is:

> the care which recognises and responds to the needs of the human spirit when faced with trauma, ill health or sadness and can include the need for meaning, for self worth, to express oneself, for faith support, perhaps for rites or prayer or sacrament, or simply for a sensitive listener. Spiritual care begins with encouraging human contact in compassionate relationship, and moves in whatever direction need requires. (2011, p.3)

They go on to suggest that spirituality is about hope and strength; trust; meaning and purpose; forgiveness; belief and faith in self, others, and for some this includes a belief in a deity/higher power; peoples' values;

love and relationships; morality; creativity and self-expression. They emphasise that spiritual care is more than religious belief and practices and is not the sole responsibility of the chaplain. It also involves:

- meeting people at the point of deepest need

- not just 'doing to' but 'being with'

- our attitudes, behaviours and our personal qualities (i.e. how we are with people)

- treating spiritual needs with the same level of attention as physical needs.

However, there is a lack of consistency in the literature and Clarke (2009) suggests that there has been a lack of critical engagement about the concept of spirituality and a tendency towards separating religion and spirituality. This has led to a broad, generic approach to spiritual care which makes it hard to explain and difficult to put into practice. One simple definition of spirituality within a paediatric context which has merit in relation to spiritual care is the 'ability of a child through relationships with others to derive personal value and empowerment' (Hart and Schneider 1997, p.263).

Chaplaincy perspectives

In some earlier writing focusing on palliative care and bereavement Paul offered a definition of spirituality as 'a lifelong journey on which people explore their connectedness to the world, themselves, others and possibly the transcendent, and the meaning and purpose of their lives; that which gives my life meaning and value' (2011, p.2). Spiritual care was described as concerning itself with the big questions of life involving who someone is, and that person's purpose, destiny, identity and potential for a relationship with the transcendent.' He also suggests that chaplains engage in spiritual, religious and pastoral care while acknowledging that these cannot always be clearly differentiated.

Child spirituality perspectives

While Eaude (2009) suggests that spirituality has its roots in religion and it is not helpful to divorce the term from its roots, others suggest that there is an innate spirituality in young children (Hay and Nye 2006; Hyde 2008). Hyde (2008) identifies three core elements in the discourse on children's spirituality. The first is a sense of search, which is about seeking answers to questions around identity, place and purpose; the second is a search for meaning, including pursuing happiness but making sense of suffering, pain and loss; the third is the notion of connectedness, which includes both independence and interdependence as well as a sense of awe and wonder. A landmark study was carried out by Hay and Nye (2006) who interviewed primary school pupils. This led them to identify the concept of relational consciousness as the core element of children's spirituality. This contains four elements: an awareness of self, others, the environment and, for some, the transcendent other.

Social work perspectives

Holloway (2006), writing in the British context, opts for an inclusive definition of spirituality, which includes both formal religious belief systems as well as non-traditional ones. However, she argues that social work has demonstrated little interest in the debate on spirituality that occurs in other helping professions. There is thus a reluctance to engage in spiritual care, which may also relate to a historical antipathy to religion in social work in the West and a desire to move away from the Christian charitable foundation of the profession. Holloway suggests that there is merit in introducing spirituality into social work practice as it would reflect some of the core values that are threatened by the market driven service delivery that is the context for many social workers today. However, within the USA, the social workers' ethical code states that spirituality must be included within assessment (Puchalski and Ferrell 2010, p.35).

Spiritual pain or distress

There are elements of the hospital experience that may cause spiritual pain or distress, which we need to be aware of as spiritual care practitioners. Although they have children and young people's best interests at heart, some of the adults who visit them may cause them pain as a consequence of necessary treatment. It also needs to be remembered that other children and young people may hear or observe this trauma, which may evoke fear that this may happen to them. Learning to trust adults who approach them may be more difficult than in other contexts. A stay in hospital means that young people have to engage with separation and loss with the potential of the grief associated with this. Some, particularly younger children, may not have the words or conceptual development to identify this as the cause of their negative feelings. It is therefore important that patients have frequent opportunities to talk and ask questions and have ways of externalising emotions. This may bring an enhanced need for comfort and reassurance. Fear can be significant and enabling patients to verbalise that fear is an important dimension for their spiritual health.

Finding ways of facilitating a peaceful environment, at least temporarily, may be particularly important. They are also moving home for a period of time, with hospital becoming the new home, and making it feel like home may be difficult. Boredom can also be a consequence of being in hospital. It is also important to appreciate the time and energy it may take parents to engage their child who is a long-term patient or for children who do not have parents there regularly, if they are not able to go to school. How do they fill their time (at least some of the time) in a way that nurtures them, as would be the case when they are not in hospital?

Conclusion

We appreciate that there is much good paediatric spiritual care happening around the world and that the discipline of spiritual care can draw on and learn from insights from other disciplines. We are mindful of the importance of focusing on the assets rather than deficits of our children and young people and are learning so much from them as we engage in spiritual care. Chapters 3 to 10 include both practice examples and activities, and we see narrative as one of the best ways of exploring spiritual care. Chapter 2 elucidates our best practice principles for spiritual care; Chapter 3 introduces the concept of interpretive spiritual encounters; Chapter 4 focuses on identity; Chapter 5 on creating spaces for spiritual care; Chapter 6 on meaning making; Chapter 7 on work with families; Chapter 8 on spiritual practices; Chapter 9 on tensions and issues; and Chapter 10 on facilitating spiritual literacy.

Chapter 2

Best Practice Principles
for Spiritual Care

The Royal College for Paediatrics and Child Health (RCPCH) established a participation project as a part of its strategy of enhancing engagement with patients. BCH took this challenge seriously and appointed a participation manager to lead on this. Two of the original objectives were to encourage participation projects within the hospital and to create a young person's advisory group (YPAG). The former proved to be an ideal vehicle for us to learn more about spiritual care with hospitalised children and young people. We thus formally undertook a participation project and the initial impetus for this book emerged from this (Nash, Darby and Nash 2013).

Principles and practices of spiritual care for sick children

These principles are evidence based and are derived from the analysis of the data from our participation project research, ongoing reflection on our practice and discussion amongst a multidisciplinary spiritual care team. It is an evolving set of principles which we revisit in the light of fresh research and experience. The principles in practice are illustrated throughout the book and Appendix 3 provides an overview.

1. Participation, empowerment and autonomy are core underpinning values of spiritual care

Participation entails sharing power with children and young people and enabling them to make choices, ask questions, express doubts, challenge, engage or withdraw as they want to. In a context where often choice is very limited, patients value being given the opportunity for autonomy, and to decide for themselves whether to take part in a particular activity. When offered an activity, children and young people should be made aware of what will be involved and the role they and the spiritual care practitioner may play. This is integral to gaining voluntary informed consent and it is good practice to see this as an ongoing process. However, there is sometimes a tension between facilitating such autonomy and knowing when further encouragement may be helpful, as engagement in a particular activity may be in their best interests. We have had families ask us to get their child involved in activities, even when they appear reluctant, as they do enjoy it in the end. It is one of those areas where professional judgement and reflective practice is important.

Participation is one of four commonly quoted professional youth work principles in England, the others being informal education, equal opportunities and empowerment. One of our areas of learning has been to integrate best practice principles from work with children and young people into our spiritual care practice. This includes the foundational principle of play work that play is necessary for healthy development and one of our innate impulses as humans. Activities we use are interspersed throughout the book and there is a separate index to them at the back of the book. For some activities there are guidance sheets for children and young people and for staff, and many of our postcards have specific questions or activities related to them, whereas others are open to explore in a variety of ways. There are samples in Appendix 2.

2. We need to create spaces for spiritual care to occur

Creating space for spiritual care to occur includes such things as an attitude of openness and acceptance, treating children and young people with respect, being fully present, listening attentively and taking them as you find them. The Zulu greeting 'sawubona' means 'I see you' but it is a deep seeing, an acknowledgement of shared humanity, and we need to create such space. As our first principle suggests, the space may feel safer for patients if we offer them choice and autonomy and gain consent on an ongoing basis. It can be helpful at times to positively create a space that was different to the one initially presented, and a fun, happy or sacred space may each be important at different times. Although creating space for encounters is a priority for spiritual care, we need to hold this in tension with a need for privacy in an environment where many people may invade space, ask questions and require a response at a time when a child or young person may not want to give one. For young people whose space has changed radically from their life at home, ways of creating safe space for spiritual support become vital. Identifying ways in which long periods of waiting or inactivity can be used for contemplation and reflection may also be useful, and spiritual care activities can transform the perception of what is possible.

It is also important to consider what places are available for spiritual care and this will in part depend on the nature of the illness and the capacity of children and young people to move around the hospital. We most often engaged in spiritual care at the bedside but sometimes in the hospital, school, our chapel or other faith rooms, or in communal spaces such as a play room or family room.

3. Spiritual care occurs within the context of relationship

While we create space for spiritual care we are also building relationships with children and young people and their families. This involves developing rapport and trust and reflecting on things such as how one demonstrates love and care, including boundaries and appropriate touch. Listening is an essential skill in spiritual care and should be both active and attentive. Active listening involves engaging with the person and responding through body language such as nodding our head or facial expressions and using simple comments such as 'I see' or 'tell me more about that'. Attentive listening means being fully present to the other person and not formulating our own responses as they speak and resisting the temptation to interrupt or tell our own story. Often in their day-to-day hospital experience a child or young person has time and space where they have little contact with others and, for some, the experience can be quite isolating and the opportunity to build relationships with staff and patients can help develop a sense of belonging.

4. Spiritual care happens in the context of family and often with family present

There are several ways that parents or other family members impact spiritual care. Positively, they may provide children with reassurance, and an activity may give parents a vocabulary or way of talking to their child about spiritual care which can be built upon. Negatively, there are some things which children may not say in front of their parents or they may reflect their parents' view rather than their own. What can be very different for sick children is that a parent may be with them nearly all the time. Some parents may sleep in the same room or stay in the family accommodation on site, or the children may be missing one of their parents who has to stay at home to care for siblings. The stress and distress that parents feel will often be picked up by sick children and thus doing some activities together which are calming, fun, stimulating or which provide a different focus from their illness can be helpful. Other areas which merit reflecting on in context is how, where and what we pray about with parents and facilitating discussion and reflection on perceptions of and attitudes to God. As chaplains we are often seen as official faith representatives and can be a focus of anger.

5. We need to connect and build on existing spirituality and, if appropriate, faith

Building on and connecting with existing spirituality and faith is important. One way of reflecting on existing spirituality and faith is identifying what lifts the spirits of children and young people and building on this. For some it is music, others art, others their games, and so on. For some people an act of spiritual care will have more meaning if it includes religious care. This can involve a range of things from using stories from the particular faith tradition (and we have a stock of story books that we use), spiritual care activities, which can be interpreted in religious ways and festival-related activities. Prayer may be an integral element of this connecting and when we come to pray with families we have a mental list of things that may be appropriate or helpful to draw on when praying. We then seek to relate this to any existing experience of prayer the patient or their family has, explain what will happen and agree whether or not the child, young person or parent will pray too. It becomes important to listen carefully and reflect concerns and priorities in any verbalised prayer. Giving an opportunity for children and young people to compose their own prayers, using various creative means, can lead to some beautiful and heartfelt expressions of prayer. Utilising a prayer tree may also be appreciated. A prayer tree is a place to hang your own prayers written on leaf-shaped paper. It may be a real tree in a pot, artificial branches or a wooden tree skeleton, for example. In many cases, children and young people welcome being prayed for but they also need the space to articulate their own prayer, to express and share from within.

6. Developmental and learning context is important to understand in choosing activities, resources and language

Understanding the context is vital in spiritual care. Sickness can impact development emotionally and psychologically, as well as physically. The young person in hospital is probably different to the young person at home and it is important to understand these differences as some of them are the source of their spiritual needs. As well as seeking to identify spiritual care needs the ability (physical and mental), location, learning styles and multiple intelligences (Gardner 1983) are all issues which may need to be considered. Gardner (1983) suggests that there are much broader ways of looking at intelligence, such as linguistic, logical-mathematical, musical, bodily-kinaesthetic, spatial, interpersonal and intrapersonal, and understanding this may help develop appropriate activities that meet the needs of different children and young people. A simple way of understanding learning styles is by using the acronym VAK – visual, auditory and kinaesthetic. Visual learners focus on seeing and reading, auditory learners on listening and speaking and kinaesthetic learners on touching and doing (for more information see Chislett and Chapman 2005–2012).

Having strategies for the severely disabled or very restricted because of their medical condition is important. There are also potential issues around literacy, language and cultural and religious beliefs. For example, an activity designed around the story of the three little pigs is not appropriate for a Muslim child. One young person, aged 14, had difficulty reading and writing. She had limited fine motor skills due to injury, and yet was fluent and articulate when given the opportunity to voice her thoughts and prayer into a digital recorder.

7. Metaphor can be a significant tool for spiritual care

Metaphor can be seen as a way of thinking (see Lakoff and Johnson 1980 for an overview) and can be used in a variety of ways to help children make connections in spiritual care. Finding books, songs, activities, and so on, which open up conversations about spiritual care issues works very well, as they are seemingly 'normal' activities but give the opportunity to explore and express emotions and reflect on experiences. Examples include using a butterfly image, a lion image, the story of the lost sheep, hearts, child held in God's hand, and 'blob' pictures. When linked with their significant hospital experience, such metaphors have the potential to go on nurturing children, long after they have left the hospital. However, careful thought needs to be given to the context and any potential dangers of using metaphor, including taking it too literally.

8. Spiritual care occurs within and by a community and can offer windows of normalisation

Community is a significant concept in spiritual care and there can be a variety of new communities to join or to form as part of the experience of being sick and hospitalised. Jason argues that:

> To attain a psychological sense of community, we should develop traditions, norms, and values that are tied to the settings or communities in which we live. The notion of a supportive community represents a comprehensive way of thinking about health and healing. Such an approach combines strategies that strengthen inner resources by instilling hope, confidence, enthusiasm, and the will to live with strategies that provide a place for people to live that is protected and nourishing. (1997, p.75)

Hospital is a new community and helping patients attain this psychological sense of community is important. It is often an ever-changing community as nurses work shifts, new patients arrive; there is little that is constant. In some ways, a new home has to be created and how we facilitate that, for example, through the personalisation of the bed space, can be important.

Finding opportunities for patients to be together, if they are well enough, is important and notions of belonging and peer support are elements which nurture our spirituality. What is related to this is the idea of windows of normalisation. Can we create opportunities for children and young people and their families to do 'normal' things together as they may do when at home? One of the chaplains facilitates a tea and cake session which replicates the sort of thing one would get at a church or voluntary organisation. Links back to their own community are also important and helping patients process the loss they feel may be part of the spiritual care task, as may be encouraging contact and visits. Activities which help children and young people talk about some of these emotions can be important. It may also be significant to help them to see that they are part of a new community which values them.

The community for spiritual care practitioners is also the multidisciplinary team. Thus, offering spiritual care as part of a multidisciplinary team provides opportunities for mutual learning between disciplines. As chaplains, we try to work alongside play, youth work, psychology, nursing, allied health professionals and medical staff. For example, the chaplaincy team have learnt from the play and youth workers about risk assessments and they have grown in understanding and confidence about offering spiritual care from the chaplains. We have also learnt the importance of supporting each other and offering spiritual care to staff alongside trying to ensure our own spiritual needs are met.

We also brought in spirituality specialists with children and young people and spiritual care experts to advise us. This was crucially done early on in development and helped us to take wider theories and best practice into account as we developed our own practice. We now offer training to multidisciplinary staff and other chaplains in paediatric spiritual care.

9. Meaning making helps children and young people articulate, identify and understand their spiritual needs

Meaning making is integral to spiritual care and can happen when one connects with what is already there, as well as through new activities. Encouraging 'show and tell' may provide opportunities for children and young people to talk about the things and relationships that are important to them by focusing on what is in and around their bed space. For example, a special toy may have been alongside the child throughout all of their treatment. Treating such a toy with respect and care becomes immensely important.

Meaning making also happens through episodes of spiritual care and it can be helpful to review these at a later date. 'Remember when' can be the start of a significant conversation, building on what has gone before and enabling children to share new thoughts or connections they have made. Marking significant moments is also a part of this, which may mean a prayer or blessing before an operation or celebrating a particular milestone along the way. Mapping or reflection exercises may help the child to notice the positive, life-enhancing parts of their experience, which are also present but may be overshadowed by the challenges. We try to give a child or young person scope to explore both the light and dark within the hospital experience: the hopes, fears and needs they may have. We may often be surprised by young people's construction of meaning, and need to avoid loading them with our expectations and assumptions.

One of the things we have tried hard to do is to identify how illness impacts the spiritual needs of children and young people, while appreciating that there are such needs common to them at particular stages of development. This includes the importance of connectedness to self, others, the world and possibly the transcendent; mystery, awe and wonder; exploring values, good and evil and what is important in life.

Thus, in our spiritual care we expect to find moments of mystery, wonder, grace and insights.

10. Identity may have a heightened significance in sickness

Identity is significant in spiritual care and may particularly become an issue when a child or young person is in hospital and is having to come to terms with a new identity as a sick person. Spiritual care involves affirming a positive identity and helping them to see who they are and how valuable, precious and special they are within this new context. Names are highly important: remembering names, calling people by their preferred names and exploring the significance of a name are all vital.

11. Concrete and visible expressions and reminders of spiritual care are important

Leaving something behind that acts as a reminder or an opportunity for ongoing reflection is one of the things that emerged as valuable from our participation project. One patient went down to theatre clutching a card with a picture of a child in God's hand. Another has a bracelet, which she wears all the time except when it might get dirty, where the beads represent different attributes she has or desires. One child received a small blanket (handmade by a volunteer), which had a picture of lions, a significant symbol of identity for him. We are developing a wide range of postcards and business-size cards that can be left or, in some instances, just picked up in chapel.

However, we need to acknowledge that not all spiritual care happens intentionally; it can happen in brief encounters in the corridor or by someone completing a prayer leaf for the tree. Most of all, what we often leave behind is who we are and how we have made someone feel (Nash, Nash and Frith 2011).

Making opportunities to showcase and share spiritual care is valuable. Around the hospital are a variety of places where activities that children and young people have completed can be displayed, including the main corridor and the chapel. We often use the school summer holiday as an opportunity to do a big project that is then displayed. We have found that for many young people this facilitates a desire or need to share with the wider hospital about how being ill and in hospital feels – it helps them to feel they are giving something back.

12. Offering 'episodes of spiritual care' reflects the often integrated nature of assessment and intervention and the element of reciprocity

While the terms 'assessment' and 'intervention' fit well within a hospital environment, and other staff readily comprehend them, they do not fully represent the process that takes place in spiritual care as they are usually seen as separate processes. What is more accurate is that when members of staff offer a child or young person an episode of spiritual care based on their knowledge and understanding of that child or young person, the episode of care provides an opportunity for the child to express spirituality. One of our most significant observations from the participation project was that assessment and intervention are integrated and that often the activity we were using as part of what we originally called the assessment was actually an intervention. The metaphor of television programmes, where there may be a one-off, short series, longer series or soap, may have something to offer in reflecting on the nature of the episodes. The term 'episode of care' would also resonate in a medical context. The notions of the intuitive practitioner (Atkinson and Claxton 2000) or mindful practice (Johns 2004) are found in reflective practice literature and we speculate that our more experienced staff are subconsciously making assessments all the time and choosing appropriate responses to them.

Conversation is a significant tool in this process (Wolfe 2001). While the practitioner may bring ideas and resources to the encounter, they are person-centred in their approach, guided by and responsive to the direction of the patient and willing to take new and unplanned routes. Hence, for example, one chaplain willingly explored all the blob pictures in a book (Wilson and Long 2009), at a young person's request, rather than merely focusing on one, as is our normal practice. The session lasted for one-and-a-half hours, an indication of the level of meaning making that was occurring. 'Episode of spiritual care' also reflects accurately the relational nature of the exchange, where the child leads the adult into realms of discovery and meaning, revealing their spiritual life, sharing their inner world. It is a regular experience that these episodes end with real, genuine and spontaneous expressions of care between the chaplain and the child. Both patient and chaplain can be inspired, moved or changed by one another.

Conclusion

We do not use one model of spiritual care but, as noted in the previous chapter, we have a working definition that we add to or revise as our learning grows, while reaffirming that spirituality is easier to explore than explain! We have developed the concept of ISE, interpretive spiritual encounters, which we explore more fully in the next chapter. It helps us to understand and interpret needs through a spiritual lens. We have learnt that assessment is ongoing, that using medical and healthcare language to explain what we do can help it to be more readily understood. We have developed these principles to ensure that we work in a safe and professional manner.

Chapter 3

Interpretive Spiritual Encounters (ISE)

PRACTICE EXAMPLE 3.1: ANOTHER BOX FOR RIA

Ria is 11, has cerebral palsy, and has spent a long time in hospital recently. She was visited by one of our spiritual care volunteers and this is her story of the encounter.

Ria has regular visits from various members of the chaplaincy team and both she and her parents are appreciative of the support. Our opening conversation was about the last time I had visited her – months ago (see Practice Example 1.1). Today we made a 'Happy Box'. Ria decorated the lid with sparkling stars then put messages and items in the box. She was delighted with the sparkle, texture and pattern she created with stars on the top of the box. Due to her cerebral palsy she finds fine motor control challenging. She occasionally asked for help but was determined to complete the design she had planned. She will look in the box when she is either happy or sad and the contents will make her smile, she said. These were the things she chose to put in the box and the messages she dictated for me to write on small pieces of card: blue glass pebble; dark smooth pebble from the beach with white lines etched through it; soft small white heart; tiny sparkling yellow flowers; small blue ribbon/bow; messages that said 'my family and me on holiday', 'Dad and me in the Disney store', 'we made this happy box for me to look in and remember today' and 'I send God's love and peace to you' (Ria asked me to write a message).

As we did this creative activity we talked together. We spoke about the journey of life being like a dark tunnel often, and light being at the end of the tunnel. As the light comes closer we are encouraged, but we spoke of God being with us in both dark and light times. She said in her experience there are often long dark tunnels but that she gets through and finds the light has come a little closer. We talked about God being with us in hard and easier times, dark and light times. She chose a black pebble with thin white lines on it to put in the box which represented these experiences. Ria also told me about her visit to Lapland a couple of years ago, where she saw the northern lights. She said no words could describe the sight. We talked of feeling part of something bigger than yourself when you see something so amazing, it's real but indescribable. She went on to say, 'I am a miracle. I was one pound and two ounces when I was born and my mum was very ill, she had septicaemia.' She then told me about a YouTube film she had watched about a miracle baby and said 'I believe in things like that. I believe in miracles.'

Amongst other things, I learnt:

- the importance of the gift of time, communicating value to a child or young person

- the positive significance of building on a past encounter, and the value of continuity in relationship and trust developing

- the deep spiritual awareness of an 11-year-old who has a life of challenge due to disability and long periods of hospitalisation

- the widely varied levels of spiritual, cognitive and physical development and the need to connect appropriately

- that hope, heaven, recognising sadness, darkness, challenge, loss are all significant on a child's spiritual journey

- the importance of process not product

- the importance of affirmation

- helping children explore their spiritual/inner world is a reciprocal experience.

Liz Bryson, spiritual care volunteer

When we came to reflect upon what was happening as we piloted our original activities, we very quickly realised that something significant was happening as we engaged in the activities with patients, as Ria's story above illustrates. An analysis of our recording sheets showed how spiritual needs were being articulated by the children and young people, and the activities did help to meet those needs. And as Ria's story also illustrates, sometimes religious care is part of spiritual care. Paul began to try to find a framework for holding these connections together. What was happening with the children? Who else was seeing what was happening as we undertook activities with the patients? Was there a term that got to the essence of what was happening when we played? This is where the concept ISE, interpretive spiritual encounter, was born. This was in 2012, and we have found that it captures the creative mutual nature of an activity as an assessment and intervention tool, which takes seriously the nature of working with and supporting children and young people.

What is an ISE?

An interpretive spiritual encounter is what we are seeking to achieve when we engage in spiritual care with children and young people. It is the significant participative nature of the encounter that creates and offers the time and space for them to explore safely spiritual needs, concerns about their health or whatever is on their mind. The power to disclose their spiritual needs, distress, journey objectives and questions, generally and specifically due to their illness or condition, lies with young people. We facilitate these encounters by offering activities that appeal to different characteristics of the patient and which are appropriate to their development levels, condition, ability and interests, including the concept of what lifts their spirits. There is intentionality in our visiting, which creates the potential for an ISE to occur while always respecting the right of a child to say 'no' or choose not to engage at all. All the words in the ISE are carefully chosen and while we could have used the word experience instead, that can be one sided. We thought that the dynamic nature of encounter was more insightful and shaping of our approach to spiritual care as it involves more than one person. It is not prescriptive of content but acknowledges the significance of the meeting.

From assessment to intervention

In discussion at our Multidisciplinary Paediatric Spiritual Care Working Group (MPSCWG) we were reflecting on our observations of something happening beyond simply doing activities. We hypothesised that not only did the activities work as an assessment resource, but also that an intervention happens during the encounter. We shared stories of how activities identified the child's needs, and as we went on those needs began to be met. While this insight was new for some of us, our psychologists explained how this regularly happened in their initial assessments. What we then reflected on together was that in doing an assessment we take time to ask the child, young person or others present questions, to offer active listening, and to respond with empathy. Thus, we are likely to affirm them and even meet some of their needs during the assessment. This made so much sense, when we thought about how we often feel better when someone has listened to us and we know we have been heard. This is an ongoing process as assessment is not a one-off activity.

An ISE is an alternative to a more traditional way of undertaking spiritual assessment and can be the first step in developing a spiritual care plan for a child young person, who we will see more than once, as well as being a meaningful one-off encounter. Our experience, backed up by some literature on spiritual assessment (McSherry and Ross 2010), is that in paediatrics a standard list of questions may not be appropriate or helpful. Children may not have the vocabulary to understand or answer the questions and they may not be nuanced enough for the breadth of contexts encountered with sick people.

Identifying spiritual needs – a multidisciplinary responsibility

One of the pieces of work we did at BCH was to audit who had the terms spiritual, spirituality and spiritual care in their job descriptions. We found that most multidisciplinary staff had something like 'holistic needs' but almost none used the word 'spiritual'. When we had the initial meetings of the MPSCWG, we discussed the existing definitions of spiritual care and everybody in the room realised that this was a part of their job. Therefore, everyone needs ways to identify what spiritual needs are.

PRACTICE EXAMPLE 3.2: FACILITATING
SPIRITUAL WELLBEING

What I appreciate the most about my job is that there is no agenda. I come in peace and purely to enjoy and spend a little time to embrace the little things that make us happy. Children and young people in hospital are not sure how to spend their time or fill the gaps between family visit, and questions from our adolescents include, 'How will I get to know anyone?' 'Will anyone like me or remember me?' 'Can I still be independent?' They have had a sudden upheaval, possibly involving loss, bereavement, even exclusion from their peer groups and social network systems. This can impair their capacity to form constructive attachments leaving them limited within hospital, and potentially vulnerable, which seriously affects the way they engage with staff or make themselves understood. A large part of my role with adolescents is to facilitate 'the discussion' while trying to normalise an activity to open the door to their spiritual wellbeing.

Jodie Cotterrell, play facilitator

Sometimes a distinction is made between spiritual screening, which may take place when taking a patient history and which includes identifying any religious faith tradition, and a more formal spiritual assessment. However, so far, we have not landed on a formal policy for undertaking spiritual assessment, but what this has done is to encourage multidisciplinary working and referrals between us. This has liberated other staff to explore spiritual care with patients, as they can offer and engage in activities with children and young people. We are also reflecting on whether we can learn something from the difference between normative and specialist play workers in relation to spiritual care. We are looking at whether some activities can be done by any staff member and referrals made to chaplains where this is appropriate or desired, or it is clear that religious care is part of what is wanted by the child or young person.

Our experience suggests that there are some activities which work well for the first encounter with a child or young person, the initial assessment. While context determines what is most appropriate, we have found that the Bead Bracelet activity, the Blob Tree and the Examen Doll (see Appendix 2) work well for the first encounter and then a spiritual care plan can begin to be developed.

How an ISE works for new patients

1. Spiritual care practitioners have their own bag of activities that reflect the spiritual care principles in Chapter 2. These include samples and explanatory laminated sheets where necessary.

2. Spiritual care practitioners introduce themselves and offer the activities to children. If the children are interested, the practitioner shows them some of the activities in their bags and lets them choose which one(s) they would like to do.

3. The practitioner then gets out the resources to do the activity and explains any finer details of how to do it, giving full permission for the children to engage with it how they wish. According to what has been chosen and the capacity of each child, the spiritual care practitioner may undertake the activity with the children or they may do it on their own.

4. While the activity is being done, the spiritual care practitioner actively listens, watches, and with discernment and permission engages with the children and young people and invites them to talk about what they have done and why they have done it like that or explore any issues arising from the activity. This is encouraging the child or young person to engage in self-assessment. Thus, because the activity is part of an assessment, the spiritual care practitioner may also offer an interpretation to be considered (making clear that this can be rejected if not accurate or able to be owned at that time). Spiritual care practitioners are professionals who are part of a multidisciplinary team, each member of which is doing assessments in his or her area of expertise.

5. The spiritual care practitioner is encouraged to make an assessment of the spiritual life and needs being expressed or discerned and also where an engagement, meeting or intervention into those needs might have already happened or may be desirable.

6. Discussion around what has been shared and observed is offered to the child, including offers of what to do with what has been shared.

7. An offer is made to the child for the practitioner to return (see below).

8. The spiritual care practitioner makes comments in the patient's notes (where this is protocol) and in the appropriate format for the

department (this can be a recording form or book or electronic feedback sheet, for example).

9. The spiritual care practitioner follows up any referrals or concerns and reflects upon further ISEs to explore.

With ongoing patients

1. The spiritual care practitioner offers to come back and visit again or suggests another team member may visit where this is appropriate.

2. If the child says yes, they offer to chat further about what the child has explored, and to bring another activity that might facilitate further deeper discussion around particular spiritual needs or interests.

3. Then as above from point 3.

Benefits of ISE

Facilitating our objectives

Our main objectives are to offer spiritual care and build trusting relationships. We have found that ISE helps us to fulfil those objectives effectively. Staff go in prepared with a range of activities to offer but are not prescriptive about whether they are used or how they are used. However, we have found that usually when an ISE is offered that gets a positive response.

Spiritual care is easier to explore than explain

This was one of our early discoveries as we ventured down this road. We wondered how we would explain to children and young people, their families and staff what we were offering and doing. How do you start to explain to 5-year-olds that we were interested in engaging with their deepest existential spiritual questions?! As we trialled the activities, we found that we did not need to explain what we were doing; we just offered the activities and let the children and young people make the connections to what was important to them at that moment.

Takes personal choice and autonomy seriously

As we have mentioned, this is a key principle of good practice in our offer of spiritual care. Because activities are offered, and choices given, the young people are always in control. This is an important aspect of their care, given how little control some young people have in relation to other assessments and interventions.

Gives a model for assessment and ongoing assessment
Going back and either offering another activity or asking children how they have further added to a previous activity has proved very helpful in moving away from the one-off assessment encounter.

It also gives a model and structure for engaging with children and young people in an appropriate developmental way. It helps staff to respond intuitively and instinctively. It may also facilitate early intervention, as we may identify an issue before it becomes a major problem. There is also the potential for identifying when a referral may be helpful.

ISE may help explore particular spiritual needs
in relation to a specific condition
Doing some of the activities and then analysing the responses may give us the capacity to see patterns or notice particularities in common with children and young people with a specific condition.

Faith development
ISE provides a useful model for engaging children and young people who have faith and belong to a particular religious tradition. Activities which are either faith-tradition specific or more generally religious can be used. This is usually the role of chaplains.

RESOURCES FOR ISE

Many of the activities we use are spread throughout the book and collated in an index, but those we used initially in our participation project are listed below to give an idea of the scope of what we do.

- Mixed bag of beads and a piece of elastic to make a 'Who loves/cares for me bracelet'. The different beads could represent anything or anyone that made the child feel loved/cared for. A variation was making a bracelet with beads representing something or someone important to the child.

- Offering a mixed bag of beads representing different emotions and states of being the child has experienced such as a blue bead for peace, a green bead for feeling safe, a yellow bead for hope, a red bead for irritation.

- Offering young people a lump of clay to make something that reminded them of a safe/peaceful space in their life (group exercise).

- Reading the book *Josh Stays in Hospital* with a child who had also stayed in hospital over Christmas.

- Making a prayer leaf for the chapel prayer tree with butterfly and heart stamps.

- Bible stories: discussing the meaning of names of people in the Bible, and of this child in particular.

- Visit to the intensive care ward, as part of a saying goodbye ritual, making the transition to going home. We went to the chapel; the child made a prayer image, 'remembering' his experience in the paediatric intensive care unit (PICU) (although he could not literally remember), and we had a short time of prayer and dedication at the altar, laying this image down, and blessing him on his journey.

- Teddy Postcard: discussing the young person's ideas about feeling cared for in hospital. At the end, we made a digital recording of the prayer, arising out of our discussion, as injuries meant she could not write.

- Blob pictures: discussion about the child's sense of identity, meaning, relationships and faith, as the pictures were examined.

- Singing with an infant in the PICU to lift her spirit and distract her from the many noises and, particularly, the sound of another baby crying.

- Godly Play story of the Parable of the Mustard Seed with two children in school. Godly play is an interactive and participative approach to storytelling that uses both symbols and words and encourages children to make connections between the story and their own experience (see www.godlyplay.co.uk).

- Godly Play story of the Good Shepherd with a child at her bedside.

- Praying for a child before an operation using a prayer card.

Developing ISEs

Some of the ways we have developed ISEs include:

- Taking existing activities and amending them, e.g. making bracelets, inspired by the oncology Beads of Courage. (Different coloured Beads of Courage are given to our oncology patients relating to specific treatments and procedures they have.)

- Existing spiritual engagement resources, e.g. Blob Tree.

- Identifying what is popular among children and young people at the time – again, making bracelets.

- Building on familiar metaphors and concepts, e.g. the elephant in the room, decorating a small elephant and naming what is not being talked about.

- Creating new resources, e.g. postcards for children and young people to read, engage with, be inspired by and draw upon. They may be visual or more text-oriented, e.g. picture of traffic lights or the well-known Footprints poem (www.footprints-inthe-sand.com) card, which finishes with the idea that when you see only one set of footprints on the sand God is carrying you.

- Creating new resources that have a hospital feel, e.g. bandage bracelets decorated with symbols, names or phrases.

- Saying 'Hi', having a conversation and seeing where it leads.

- Using stories, including those with cultural or religious resonance.

- Identifying a need and devising an activity to meet it, e.g. comfort or happy boxes.

- Looking at resources catalogues for children and young people and working out what could be adapted or developed, e.g. festival-related art and craft activities.

Another dimension of developing ISEs may be to take into account Csinos and Bellous' (2009) spiritual styles, which suggests that we may be word-, emotion-, symbol- or action-centred. These correspond to intellect, emotions, mystery and action. Discerning what a child or young person may be most drawn to can be helpful in choosing activities. Noting whether a deductive or inductive approach for a particular individual would be preferable may also be significant in developing an ISE.

Why ISE works

An ISE is more than doing activities, it is intentionally creating an opportunity for young people to engage with how they are feeling about their condition and situation, or other issues and concerns. An ISE is the objective; play and engagement is the means to that end. It creates a safe place for spiritual needs to be explored, conversations to be had, symbols or mysteries perhaps to be explored and moments of wonder to be evoked, for example. Thus, one of the lessons we quickly learnt was that doing the activities gave time for conversations. 'How are you today?' might open the flood gates for a child or young person to open up and talk, but more often than not it can result in a very short answer. But playing with a child creates space and time for relationships to develop, trust to be built and a safe and sometimes sacred space to explore what is important to them.

ACTIVITY 3.1: DREAM JAR

I draw a simple picture of an empty jar, and through general conversation myself and the children and young people find common interests to talk about and then add whatever they want to the picture. On one occasion, Samantha used so many colours. No specific picture or letters, just a very clever shading of bright to really dark colours. When I asked her why she used so many, her reply was that simply she loved all colours and wanted to use as many as she could, because normally she has a specific project or task that meant use of specific colours. She appreciated an opportunity just to 'go with how she felt'. She then said that her blended colours showed her confusion in her current situation. So from this assessment and intervention I was able to support her by easing her fears of the institutional chaos of the ward round. She knows her medical condition well and understands what is expected of her, but felt that one minute she was treated too much like a grown-up and taking responsibility for her medical wellbeing, but that emotionally she can't make mistakes like her friends do. I have helped her build resilience by looking back at how she has already coped.

Jodie Cotterrell, play facilitator

Meeting generic spiritual needs

One of the great things about ISE is that it can be engaged with at whatever level young people wish. Two of the issues which we hear a lot from children and young people are boredom and a lack of privacy. Initially, an ISE may be attractive as it ameliorates boredom, and privacy is significant in terms of the capacity to choose how much and what to disclose, if anything. It gives control back to the child in an area where there is not necessarily a lot.

Interpretation: 360 degrees

One of the most important principles of ISE is that everybody involved can interpret what happens to facilitate the spiritual care of children and young people. We have found that when we 'listen' to children, through their words, what they make, what they don't say, what they draw, they are exploring their spiritual needs. However, the child's own interpretation is paramount, and asking open-ended questions to explore is much more appropriate than seeking to impose our own interpretation or making assumptions about what is presented.

Spiritual play

Spiritual play is a concept we are exploring. We are seeking to explain to patients, their families and staff using familiar terms what we are seeking to offer. We do not want to be confused with other play staff, but we also want to explain that our spiritual play activities have a contextual purpose that is different to those of other play workers. It is important to remember what play does to us; it 'cuts through our self-centredness… when playing, who the children genuinely are emerges' (Grossoehme 1999, p.10).

Never underestimate the merits of a conversation

Although what we have developed in our work has been activities, if the objective is important, that is, to engage young people in their spiritual concerns and needs, then having a conversation with a child or young person is a wonderfully simple tool. We discuss spiritual conversations further in Chapter 10.

Recording and analysis

To capture what has happened in an ISE we have learnt to take notes and reflect during and shortly after the encounter to ensure that nothing is lost. When we are doing a formal participation project we use a proforma to record and interpret our interactions. We also used a multidisciplinary team to analyse the recording forms when we wrote up the report, in order to ensure a broad perspective underpinned our findings.

Reciprocity

This comes out several times in the BBC 2 series on our chaplaincy work, *Children's Hospital: The Chaplains* (2014). Several of the chaplains are seen to comment, after interactions with the children and their families, on how they have been affected by the encounter. We think this is a positive consequence of our work, as it demonstrates how spiritual care givers are committed to being lifelong learners, who go in with a mentality of not having all the answers. Although we do not seek to have our own spiritual needs met, because of the significance of the encounter, we are inspired and grow through what we are a part of.

Partnerships in developing ISEs

Co-working with the play and youthwork team in our hospital has been an exciting consequence of our chaplaincy team going down this route. When they heard us say what we were doing, they pointed out, 'But that's what we do, but we call it something different.' This was the beginning of a great synergy of disciplines in joint ventures. They clearly had the skills in play and engaging with children and young people, but were not sure about spiritual care. Because of the success of our partnership with the play and youthwork department, we went to our hospital charities for a request for funds to run a joint activity for the children and young people every school holiday. The activity would share with and inform the wider hospital community by being exhibited in our designated space. So far, we have done three projects: a 3D Blob Tree, Elephants in the Room (decopatch elephants in shoe boxes) and Dream Space canvases. These joint projects were funded by BCH charities and have been well received by children and young people and the wider hospital community.

One of the needs identified in developing skills in spiritual care was relevant training. We ran our first module focusing on multidisciplinary spiritual care in autumn 2014. As part of that we tested ISEs and encouraged students to test it out in their own context as well as at BCH. Practice Example 4.1 is an example of this. Our original discovery and development of this concept was found in running a participation project, and we have continued to run focused participation days around these values and practices, and now open them up to visitors so they can experience what we do.

Summary

Interpretive spiritual encounters:

- create space and opportunity for conversations
- provide opportunities to build trusting relationships
- facilitate the identification and exploration of spiritual needs
- act as both an assessment and an intervention.

ISE gives us a model to work to and if an ISE is the objective, how we achieve it is an evolving, endless list. We always like the story which highlights the difference between 'I just met the most important person in the world' and 'I just met someone who made me feel as if I were the most important person in the world'. We hope that ISE facilitates the latter!

Conclusion

This is an area where we plan to do further research and we want to test these activities for their validity and reliability and to become more aware of which activities facilitate the exploration of specific needs. This will help ensure ISE and the activities we use are safe and will achieve the outcomes we hope for, without being prescriptive. We also want to have a clearer idea of how ISE relates to specific contexts and illnesses.

Chapter 4

Spiritual Care, Illness and Identity

PRACTICE EXAMPLE 4.1: JANINE'S STORY

Sixteen-year-old Janine was diagnosed with a malignant tumour. Surgery and chemotherapy caused chronic weakness and fatigue and necessitated numerous hospital admissions, isolating her from school and peers. Spiritual care was offered by a liaison nurse for the 12-month period between diagnosis and death, and this is her account of that relationship. Janine found coming to terms with her diagnosis and adhering to treatment difficult; it was more important to her to fit in with peers and have minimal disruption to her lifestyle. Her initial reaction was to dye her hair pink and attend her school prom before starting treatment. We discussed how she saw herself and thought others saw her, negotiating the present and planning for the future. Initially she experienced shock and fear when she realised hair loss would occur, so colouring her hair was a way to manage her outward manifestation of her identity. Janine decided to wear a bandana.

Janine was questioning the meaning of life. Why me? Why now? I allowed time to address these spiritual concerns which contributed to her sense of wellbeing and quality of life. Fear was significant at this time and addressing fear is an important dimension of spiritual health. Janine was able to verbalise her fears in a peaceful environment, which was important. We reflected together on her existing spirituality, identifying what lifted her spirits, revealing that to be music, fashion and two friends. A crucifix necklace given to her by a friend had great symbolic meaning to her of a recent school trip. Janine chose to engage with guitar tuition, which helped her express herself and her emotions; she described music as reducing her anxieties and allowing her to feel calm and a 'normal' thing for her to do. The tutor was not medical and she found this relationship helpful. Fluctuating between mature and childlike behaviours was common; I was adaptable to fluctuations in Janine's behaviour to ensure interactions were successful, adjusting my communication to individual situations.

Janine appeared to have formed an identity in childhood that became important during adolescence, as a protector for her brother. However, once she was unable to support him whilst having her treatments, this caused a breakdown in their relationship. Janine was forming her adult identity, assimilating both her adolescent identity and her cancer identity, negotiating the present and planning for the future. Janine was given a terminal diagnosis and returned to behaviours displayed at diagnosis, the risk-taking behaviour expected for this age group. She immediately had a tattoo, socialised, was drinking alcohol and reintegrated with her peers. She attended school whenever she felt well enough. Janine planned her funeral with friends and was buried wearing bracelets made as a spiritual care activity containing the names of her peers.

My role is to understand the unique qualities of this age group – the shared norms, attitudes, and beliefs that determine their identity and behaviour, as well as the unique stresses they face on a day-to-day basis. Identifying patients' stage of identity formation and their social and developmental histories is also part of the role. Adolescents have typical concerns about being comfortable with who they are and who they want to become. They need to be allowed to mature through their illness and develop a sense of self. This can, however, be confounded by restrictions and limitations placed on them by their disease and treatment. My task is to undertake psychosocial and behavioural interventions: to assist in retaining or returning to function in significant social roles, such as child, sibling, parent, student, worker or friend, thus enabling these young people to overcome the negative impact of a health crisis and strengthen their innermost and external coping resources.

Lorraine Beddard, teenage and young adult liaison nurse

Identity is integral to what it means to be human and is an essential concept to explore in relation to sickness. We understand identity to be contextual and fluid and

> both an assertion of who we view ourselves to be and who we would one day like to become. Identity is what each of us discovers and creates in telling our story, both to ourselves and to others. But where does identity come from? It comes both from ourselves and our context. Identity is intertwined with the individual's understanding of the goals, values, and beliefs of the society in which one has been raised. Yet, it also is developed by the individual. (Jacober 2014, p.97)

If we ask how illness might affect children and young people, identity, how they see themselves might be the first aspect that comes to mind. Our work supporting children and young people in hospital confirms this. When we talk about identity we mean such things as:

- how they see themselves

- how they think other people see them

- what they are not able to do because of their illness

- how illness or injury may affect their future, job options, etc.

- I am… What adjectives do they use to describe themselves, and how many are related to their illness?

A positive view of themselves and an identity that is respected is one of six points that The Children's Society has identified as being important for improving children's wellbeing. Elements of this include:

- being comfortable with their appearance

- being physically and mentally healthy

- being respected and valued for who they are.

(Children's Society 2014)

This suggests that being aware of identity issues in relation to sickness may be particularly significant, as appearance is sometimes impacted by illness. This may be important when working with young people, as Erikson's (1995) psychosocial theory suggests that a growing sense of identity, of who we are and what our role is, forms part of early adolescent development. This developmental stage is associated with identity confusion, identity resolution and the influence of peer groups.

So, what have we discovered about identity and illness, injury and disability in children and young people?

New identity as a sick person

We have found it helpful to develop our own understanding of what it means to be human which we describe as to love and to be loved. This means that any issues relating to identity come from this starting place, which does not change through sickness, and we talk about this to parents of premature babies who have sadly died and at funerals of babies.

However, broader issues of identity may particularly become an issue when a child is in hospital, with some having to come to terms with a new identity as a sick person. With much of who we are being bound up in what we do and can do, then being ill can only impact upon this. Many children and young people have hobbies, interests, do things to amuse themselves, belong to activity and interest clubs and groups, and their ability to participate, therefore, is limited by their illness. One of the stories that has influenced our approach to practice is of a young child in a wheelchair who is overcome one day when someone in a shop talks to him rather than to his mum. His response was, 'Mummy, he thinks I am real!' It is so important to engage with the children and young people in their own right, not just mediate through their parents.

Labelling

'You are unique' – exploring their positive uniqueness with a child or young person is one of the greatest privileges in offering spiritual care. Thus, spiritual care involves affirming a positive identity for children or young people and helping them to see who they are and how valuable, precious and special they are within this new context. Reinforcing their significance is vital and it may be important to help them explore some of the fears and concerns they have over this. It may be that for some their fears and concerns have a basis in their actual experience. Part of what we may need to do in spiritual care is challenge some of the unhelpful labelling that does go on, or the tendency to describe people in terms of characteristics that do not enhance their identity positively.

Because of the distinctive nature of paediatrics, we are sometimes trying to affirm uniqueness for the parents more than the child. One example of this is the beautiful handmade (by one of our volunteers) blankets that we offer. One was bright red and white and the chaplain observed it looked more like a cape, and so the nickname Super Stan was coined for the baby. Sometimes when you are talking directly to children, ostensibly offering spiritual care to them, it may also involve vicarious spiritual care for others at the bedside, as they are also comforted by the words.

ACTIVITY 4.1: WHAT IS IMPORTANT TO YOU?

We have a postcard that asks the question, 'What is important to you?' We have found this card useful as it not only asks an open question, it also communicates that another adult is interested in them, their needs and their views. When we did it on A3 sheets in the school, we got a wonderful array of answers. Many of the students referred to music, sport and their family. Some wrote 'to be cared for' and 'to be loved'.

I am my social media presence

Young people may have multiple identities, some of which may be on social media. Dilemmas may arise for them if they are too ill to post or if their situation means that there is nothing of interest to post, or if their posts about their illness do not get the response they would hope for. Identity can be influenced by how others respond to what we put out there.

I am my celebrity status

With a high level of media interest sometimes in showing brave, sick children and their families on TV, some may find it enhances self-image to have the cameras on them but there can be a danger of how a child or young person feels when the attention is no longer there. We have seen both these situations occur among those with whom we have worked.

PRACTICE EXAMPLE 4.2: LIZZIE'S BEADS
– WHAT'S IMPORTANT IN LIFE

Lizzie (7) was offered the bead-making activity as a focus for reflecting on the important people and things in her life. In this instance, the chaplain had already developed a relationship with Lizzie and her family and was aware that Lizzie liked to have people around her. As a result of an inoperable tumour, Lizzie had limited mobility and long periods of treatment in hospital, separated sometimes from her two siblings and one of her parents. The disruption to family life was keenly felt. In addition, Lizzie who had once enjoyed being active, was essentially paralysed. Being physically limited and almost entirely reliant on others was having an impact, yet Lizzie had a strong sense of herself in relation to those she was close to and felt secure within her family. She had also established strong bonds with some of the hospital staff.

While the chaplain had to make the bracelet for Lizzie, Lizzie chose each bead and the order in which they came. Though interrupted a couple of times by other professionals making their rounds, this did not detract from the experience, as they expressed interest and affirmed what Lizzie was doing. Lizzie started with her immediate family but went on to include wider family, her favourite nurse and physiotherapist, as well as two favourite holiday destinations, a favourite activity of drawing and family nights. Lizzie remained engaged and enthusiastic throughout the activity, and in relation to the 'place beads' told stories of family holidays and the wild risk-taking activities she loves. It was significant that a physiotherapist received special mention, as Lizzie had been reluctant to engage with physiotherapy in the fear that movement might not return. Each bead on her bracelet represented something important to Lizzie, the person, rather than Lizzie, the patient.

Rev Rachel Hill-Brown, chaplain

Names

Our experience suggests that names are highly important and we should use people's names and draw on their meaning, connections and significance where appropriate. This may involve us in asking questions around why a particular name was chosen or doing some research on the name.

PRACTICE EXAMPLE 4.3: HEAVEN BACKWARDS

Working in a hospital as a person with dyslexia, name badges are a gift! If I had my way I would get staff to write them out phonetically as well, to at least give me a fighting chance of not only remembering it but also pronouncing it! We had a very poorly baby with one of these unusual names and I was the named chaplain for the intensive care unit that day, and the staff member who came to give us the referral explained how important the name and the pronunciation was to them: Nevaeh. It was a name I had not come across before, but have many times since. So the support staff and I sat down for me to figure out how to pronounce the name and how I could remember it. My normal strategy is to write it out as I would say it, so we went with Nev vay er! After more than a little practice and trepidation, I went to visit the family. I said hello to the family, introduced myself and asked how Nev vay er was. The family was taken aback, and quickly told me I was the first member of staff to pronounce it correctly! This set the platform for a significant supportive relationship, as Nevaeh got worse and eventually died. The family told me their invitation for me to do the funeral was on the basis that they knew I would correctly pronounce the name of their gift from heaven.

Rev Paul Nash, chaplain

Spiritual care can give the opportunity to contribute

One of the early insights we received in undertaking our multidisciplinary spiritual care activities was when we gave the children and young people the opportunity to contribute to an exhibition of their activities. In many ways, such things are normalising activities, as producing something to take home or display is a regular part of childhood experience. It gives both the children and their parents something to be proud of. Thus, around the hospital there are display cases showing the work of young people. Also, some of the spiritual care activities involve making things which can be used as gifts for family or friends.

Whole family impact

Sickness can be viewed as an intrusion into what childhood should be, and it can be distressing for the family as a whole; the identity of siblings and parents may also be impacted. In some cases, engaging with the whole family may be the most important thing, as that is where a significant element of identity comes from. It may be that while in hospital the sense of being a family needs nurturing, particularly if there are siblings too.

Because of the nature of paediatrics, the children have more contact with their parents than they would at home. The lives of parents can therefore revolve around the care of their child. When this becomes the role of the family, the identity of parents can change, in how they view themselves and how they are viewed and/or referred to. For example, 'That's the family with a child with cancer.' This can also be reflected in how the siblings of ill children and young people see themselves, 'That's Ben's brother, you know, the one who was hit by a car.'

Many of our larger children's hospitals will have their own school and we are fortunate to have a great relationship with our James Brindley School. When we go in to explore spiritual wellbeing or religious celebrations, we can often find there are more siblings than patients in the school, as many of the children and young people are too incapacitated to leave their bed or their ward. Most of these siblings seem to be there because the families are not able to juggle getting them to their own schools and being there for their hospitalised child's treatments, particularly because we are a regional as well as a local hospital. Most of the siblings I have met are very proud of how their siblings are handling their illness and treatments. But what of their identity, what or who is their life revolving around, whose needs are perhaps subconsciously being prioritised? Many of the activities we use focus upon how important, loved and listened to the child is. As we think about the distinct needs of siblings, let us be mindful in our encounters of their potential, unique needs, including affirmation of who they are, and the importance of their needs.

As we have mentioned, the life of a family can revolve so much around caring for an ill child, it is understandable that when their child goes home there may be some adjustments to make. Doing activities with families can be a great way to engage with these potential issues of identity. Through conversations about normalising and finding a new normal, families can be encouraged find a new identity.

PRACTICE EXAMPLE 4.4: MARIGOLD'S FAMILY

We have a postcard which has a traffic light on it and some questions on the back to help you reflect on what areas in your life are red, amber or green. Mum was in hospital with her toddler and also had three other adolescent children who were with Dad at home. In this case, the mum was going to do the traffic light cards with the other member of the family having done them herself with the chaplaincy volunteer. They chatted about the way we all have to 'stop' doing certain things/bad habits/negative ways of thinking; 'get ready' for challenges, which for the girls may be difficult news regarding their sister; and 'go' – things that she wanted God to grow and develop in the girls. Mum was thrilled to take these cards to give to the girls for them to each fill in personally in their own time. Although this is a spiritual care card, the opportunity was there to talk about God, because for this family spiritual care also has a religious care dimension too. One of the encouraging things that we can do is facilitate family members to offer spiritual care to other members of their family.

Liz Bryson, spiritual care volunteer

Exploring identity

Spiritual care gives us the opportunity to develop a child or young person's positive identity, as it can focus on who they are as people, not just on what they can do. As with many aspects of spiritual wellbeing and care, identity is also connected to other aspects. Children's identities can be in their ability or skills, and they may already have hopes and dreams about their future.

PRACTICE EXAMPLE 4.5: GEORGE'S STORY

George (13) had leukaemia, and when I first knew him he had had a bone marrow transplant and was having fortnightly treatments at BCH. One of the side effects George faced was very fragile skin. This was not helpful as George was interested in and good at cooking. George was a referral from one of the psychologists who was supporting the family and knew I used to be a chef. The psychologist thought it could be good for George to talk to someone who could encourage and share his interests. I spent some time talking with George about cooking. I seemed to gain some credibility for my four years as a chef at the Savoy and Dorchester in London. Because of the condition of George's hands it was speculative as to whether he would be able to work in such an environment. Unbeknown to George, I thought it might be a rewarding experience for George to visit the kitchens of our hospital. On reflection, I think not only that I wanted to do this nice thing for George, but also that I was inspired by the example of organisations that are set up to help dreams come true for people with life-limiting illnesses. I discussed the possibility of George's visit with the catering manager, Tony. He was very accommodating and said he would do all he could to make this happen. I mentioned it to George's family, and then to George – he was so excited! So the momentous day came but George was ill. We rearranged it and some of his family joined us. Tony and the team were great with him. Tony introduced himself to George and explained that they did not do free tours of the kitchen and he would have to do some cooking first with two of the senior chefs. George's eyes lit up and his whole body lifted. He also explained that he was not suitably dressed. Tony brought out a jacket with George's name embroidered on it! This I think was spiritual care. I was seeking to bring a sense of meaning to George's life, to give him a 'wow' type moment and for him to experience something he could do that was fun and fulfilling. I sought to bring appropriate hope to George, affirm his gifts and abilities, engage with his interests, values and questions concerned with his unique life and journey.

Rev Paul Nash, chaplain

Other dimensions of identity may also be impacted. For example, some diseases, such as renal disease, may cause developmental delays which can impact sexual identity, and hereditary or genetic disease can also have issues which impact identity.

Illness can affect rites of passage

Within many worldviews, there are occasions that mark the change of status of a child to young person or adult. Several world religions have these for children and young people and it is important to note, not only how these might happen in hospital, but how illness might affect them.

For instance, within Islam, children and young people are expected to fulfil their adult religious requirements, not according to their age, but according to when they reach puberty. This is difficult enough to support appropriately in hospital, but what about the diseases that slow down puberty? How might these affect the identity and wellbeing of a child or young person in hospital? (See Nash, Parkes and Hussain 2015 for further details about how faith may influence care.)

Religious identity

For some of our young people and families their religious affiliation and identify is integral to their wellbeing in hospital, as it is for the whole of their lives. At the time of writing, our hospital has a population of about 9 per cent Roman Catholics. One young person aged about 15 is a regular visitor to our hospital for various lengths of stay. She identifies herself as a Roman Catholic. If she is in for more than a week, she will ask the nurses to request that our Roman Catholic chaplain brings her communion. Mum wants her daughter to have the same religious support in hospital that she has when she is at home or school.

PRACTICE EXAMPLE 4.6: PRAYING WITH JACK

One day I bumped into a young person, Jack, and his mum who was pushing him in his wheelchair towards their physiotherapy appointment. For many months Jack (13) had been unable to speak after a car accident had caused him brain damage. He had begun to make sounds, which had been a tremendous encouragement to his mum who has been alongside him, day and night, soothing, comforting, encouraging and gently challenging him in his recovery. After a long period of being lost and distressed inside a silent suffering place, he began to emerge with a new and bright spirit. He began to use an alphabet chart to spell words for others, showing immense patience with this laborious process of communication. A sports enthusiast, Jack's perseverance and courage were inspiring and I had suggested during his recovery that it was as if he was engaged in a long marathon or was conquering a high mountain and should be given a medal to celebrate his physical achievement. At the end of our conversation he pointed to my dog collar. 'Yes,' said his mum, 'she is a chaplain.' Jack spelled out 'p-r-a-y-e-r' and then brought his hands together and looked at me expectantly.

I was taken aback by his humility and the expression of openness on his face and sought words to express a prayer that might hold some meaning and truth for him. Although I might have been searching to find words, when I lifted my own eyes again he was grinning at me and his arm reached out to embrace me with happy warmth and enthusiasm. His mum looked as pleased as Jack as they carried on in the direction of their physiotherapy session.

Rev Kathryn Darby, chaplain

Who am I to God?

Within the Christian faith, one of the essential aspects that we stress is that we are unconditionally loved by God. We explain, because Jesus died on a cross, that we have a wounded Jesus who cares for and prays for us. This helps us to explore with people how they are made in the image of God. This is not an easy concept to explore, but for those children and young people who have a belief and trust in God for their lives and illness, it is essential that this is addressed, so that they see themselves as beautiful in the eyes of God.

ACTIVITY 4.2: GOD'S DAISY

This is one of our postcards that gets some of the most 'ahhh' responses. It uses the image of the child's game of picking petals one by one with 's/he loves me, s/he loves me not'. The picture on the postcard is of a daisy with only one petal left on it, with the caption, 'start with he loves me'. Most of us have put this card away when we have sensed that a child needed to be affirmed in their God's love for them, particularly if they have been in a low place over 'how can God love me, if this has happened to me?'

One of the helpful conversations we have with one of our atheist consultants is about when children get to choose their own religious affiliation. It is a helpful point for us not to assume a religious identity of a child or young person just because the parents have one and vice versa. There may also be a range of different religious identities within the family. Our definition of spiritual care includes the potential of a relationship with God/the transcendent, therefore this is reflected in the nature of our spiritual care activities. Most of them are designed to engage with belief and God only if the child or young person mentions it.

Transition: temporary and permanent nature of our patients

In a research project we undertook with young people who have cancer and their families we explored how transition was affected by illness (Darby, Nash and Nash 2014a, 2014b). Transition is both a natural part of child development stages and a term we use when our teenage patients begin to move to adult services. What we noted was that the young people were naturally transitioning through adolescence to early adulthood, growing in independence and autonomy. However, due to their illness and aggressive treatments and how ill this made them feel, they would be turning to their parents for more support, spending more time with them and relying on them more than their natural development body and mental clock might suggest would be the case. This sense and image of going in different directions encouraged us to see this process as 'inverted transition': one part of the young person with cancer is growing away from parents, and another is pushing them back.

Pushing boundaries

This is a natural process in child and adolescent development which can be difficult to manage in a hospital or hospice environment. A common issue is non-compliance in taking/having treatments and medicines. Our hospital did one of its weekly grand round presentations on a case like this. The young person was declining all interventions and did not seem to worry if she deteriorated or even died. The consultant at the end of the discussion reflected, 'I wonder what would have happened if I had taken an hour to listen to her at the beginning of the diagnosis.' The need for safe risk taking is essential to develop a healthy self-identity and image. I imagine that some non-compliance is because these children and young people have so little control over many aspects of their lives, that they take control where they can.

PRACTICE EXAMPLE 4.7: WORKING WITH ZACH

Zach (15) was hugely into sport; sport was his life and future, and main interest. Suddenly that option is gone and the questioning starts: 'Who am I? What do I do without it? Cancer – I can't ignore it, but it is not all that defines me; I have to search for a new identity – there is more to me than this. The cancer episode is an important chapter of my life, but it is not everything.'

Some of the key issues for spiritual care:

- The sense of identity is so skewed; all that defined the children and young people previously suddenly gets turned upside down: lifestyle, hobbies, friends – as they are thrown into a different world.

- Many young people will say that although they did not wish it, they would not delete this chapter from their life, given the chance. 'I would not be who I am now without it.' They would still want that part of the journey with them, even when they have lost people, friends, to cancer.

- There can be a danger of not moving on from that person-with-cancer identity – or from someone who has survived, or lived with cancer. There can be almost a 'celebrity status', which can also be something that is difficult to move on from.

- They mature so quickly; they have looked death in the eye and have been changed by the experience; they are not the same, they cannot return to where they were with friends. But at the same time, they can be immature – they have missed certain social interactions and stages.

- It is important to help young people move away from the cancer experience – it's always there, and an important part of them, but not everything that they are.

Zoe Allton, oncology youth support worker

What we have in common

Another dimension of spiritual care is to seek to build solidarity between patients with similar conditions. For children and young people to meet and hear the stories of others in similar situations can be both educative and liberating. However, there may be some situations where this is not helpful, for example where young people who self-harm have shared stories of how to harm themselves and not be discovered.

ACTIVITY 4.3: BEING A JOURNALIST

One of the things we are interested in finding out is, 'What is the difference between being at home and in hospital?' and we tried an activity that sought to discover this. Our hope was to get material for an online article and we worked in the secondary part of the school with five patients aged 13 to 16. I took along two of our microphones from the chaplaincy store room and invited the young people to interview each other. A few of them worked out what questions they would ask and who was going to be the interviewer and interviewee. As you can imagine, some of them took it more seriously than others. They enjoyed playing around with the mics, almost thrusting them up each other noses when asking their questions. Some of the things that were heard were:

> 'The thing is in hospital, they want to know every time you go for a pee.'

> 'There is so much less to do in hospital than at home.'

When those who wanted to had taken it in turns, we looked at what they might write in their article. There was a quick consensus that 'it was more boring and they had less privacy in hospital than they had at home'. It was short article! One of the things that struck us as we did this activity was the passion and fervency in their voices as they answered the questions; there was real power and conviction. This was especially noticeable from one of the girls who we knew well. She was normally so patient and gentle. During this activity, she found her voice and let rip about having to tell the nurses about her toilet habits.

Rev Paul Nash, chaplain

This activity can tell us much about the need for adolescents to have their own boundaries, to keep some things private and to be given the opportunity to share what they think and let their voice be heard.

Vicarious patients

For some young people it is very difficult to share their own needs, so that finding ways of helping them to talk may be useful. This may be through a 'vicarious' patient such as a puppet, teddy bear or other soft toy.

ACTIVITY 4.4: TEDDY GOES TO HOSPITAL

We have designed an A5 card with a picture of a bandaged teddy on it and a series of questions about how teddy feels about their experience. It gives the opportunity to start a conversation but also to then ask some follow-up questions as well such as 'Do you ever feel like that?' if it seems appropriate. Sometimes it is really clear that the children realise they are talking about themselves but, again, developmental issues will influence this. What it does accomplish is that the child is able to express some feelings and experiences in a safer way.

Conclusion

During illness, we might expect difficult feelings to emerge, both in the children and within ourselves as care givers. Effective spiritual care will not shy away from these aspects of identity, while also recognising that the handling of difficult material requires sensitivity and ongoing self-reflection and development as a practitioner. What becomes important is noticing the complexity of a child's feelings, and the complexity of our own feelings in response.

Summary

- Always refer to patients as more than their illness.

- Commit ourselves to see the child or young person as a fully whole human.

- Affirm every child and young person as being a beautiful, unique human being.

- Respect the identity that the individual is owning for themselves while challenging any destructive elements of this.

Chapter 5

Creating Spaces for Spiritual Care

Introduction

Children and young people need space to grow, and given optimum conditions, they will thrive. In attending to their spirits and bodies, we bring awareness as spiritual care practitioners of this need to facilitate the space for them to grow, a particularly important concern in a busy hospital environment where many children are living together with family members in a confined space. Human beings are very adaptable and, like plants, will strive to grow even in unlikely circumstances and surroundings. Within a hospital environment, even when the comforts of home are lacking, a child or young person will adapt and try to make the best of things.

Chaplains and spiritual care practitioners can help to create safe spaces – and sacred spaces too – which support growth by communicating the value and worth of an individual, where people feel sheltered, nurtured, upheld and encouraged to be themselves and to experience recovery. Sacred spaces can be understood as the 'in-between' that flows from one person to another, or relational spaces, where we become more aware of one another and our life with God or the world around us. Such spaces are also about an inner expansion that can come when a person is given time, attention and respect. While we work in an institution that is concerned primarily with physical health, spiritual care involves a recognition that our physicality is bound up with our emotional and spiritual life, intricately interlinked to make us the people that we are.

PRACTICE EXAMPLE 5.1: OMAR'S SNOWBALL FIGHT

Omar (5) had been on the intensive care unit for many weeks; at times, awake, aware and mobile. There were long times of boredom and frustration, and as a play worker it was important to see how his wellbeing could be enhanced. One activity involved making a special box on a pirate theme, which absorbed his interest and where he could keep special things such as pictures of his parents and a chocolate gold coin, which he could eat when he was better. The second activity was much more adventurous. I arranged for Omar to go out for a snowball fight – carefully escorted by doctors, and dressing up warm. This saw a real lift in his mood. Other medical staff engaged with Omar as a little boy first and a patient second. Having a snow ball fight, a 'normal' activity, helped humanise the situation for all. Staff became more aware that it was important to be able to get away from a confining space where possible, as that led to a low mood and a negative spirit. We arranged for Omar to go to a play room on another ward as well as spend time in the parents' room with his family.

Sally Roberts, family support play worker

Creating safe space for spiritual care

Children and young people can feel small and vulnerable particularly when surrounded by a group of adult professionals or when they are sick and away from home. Spiritual care practitioners can provide a reassuring presence and give children an increased sense of their value and worth. Creating space is about noticing the uniqueness of each young person and also about offering the growing ground for positive identity to be discovered and affirmed, by offering our loving attention and care. When invited to write a message on a stone as part of an Easter garden, one adolescent wrote, 'We are like flowers, beautiful but delicate.' A safe space begins with a listening, attentive attitude, being open, non-judgemental and accepting, and fully present to an individual. It also includes showing respect that signals to young people that they are valued, and truly heard and taken seriously. Fruitful encounters are not necessarily chatty ones; silences and reflective spaces are often the ground for spiritual growth.

When approaching a child or young person who has suffered trauma, an assessment must be made: how can I begin to create a safe space with this person, how can I help this person to build again and to recover? Just as there may be physical wounds that need time to heal, what are the appropriate kinds of support that can be offered to soothe emotional and spiritual wounds? Building trust takes time. Offering spiritual care activities can be a non-threatening way of coming alongside and getting to know a child or young person. Rather than just talking, the focus is on creating something, using colour, form, materials. At the same time, the children have company – they are not alone with all that they may be thinking or feeling, or all that has happened, perhaps having endured traumatic experiences, and they have the opportunity to share what they are going through. Engaging in the activities, the spiritual care practitioner will enjoy the company of the children and young people, as well as the creative process, and will affirm and celebrate who that person is, building esteem, giving comfort, soothing a sorrowful or wounded spirit, learning and receiving insight from the young people. Having fun is an aspect of spiritual care – it restores hope and touches on joy – which helps to address the inner balance, where distress, fear and anxiety may have taken a stronghold. Laughter and being silly sometimes, even when there is pain and anguish, can have a healing effect. Sister Florence, one of our Roman Catholic chaplains, was supporting one of our seriously ill patients, Emer, going through a difficult time after a second liver transplant. She was regularly joking and laughing with Emer, lifting her spirits. She soon got the nickname, Sister Smiley and was given a gift with this written on after Emer had recovered. Parents or carers will also relax as they see their child relaxing, and this too will have a positive impact, allowing the child who may have been aware of the parents' anxiety to feel a little more secure.

Conversations with children and young people are an important starting point for assessing where they are at and building on their existing spiritual or faith experiences, but these do not always materialise in the ways that adult conversations develop. More likely, when spiritual care practitioners get alongside a child and begin to engage with that child using visual and tactile props, opening up stories and spaces, finding other ways of listening and relating, they will find themselves drawn into a relationship with a child who is frequently open, transparent and generous in sharing thoughts and feelings.

ACTIVITY 5.1: SINGING AND DANCING – FUN AS SPIRITUAL CARE

Sometimes with a child, spiritual care is about facilitating fun, which can act as a distraction or relief. In this episode I took the role of the entertainer/clown or singing, dancing chaplain as I sometimes call this role. Alicia (7) is a small bowel transplant recipient. She is officially Church of England, and over the years most of the care has been the pastoral support of the family.

When Alicia's breathing became severely compromised, she was admitted to PICU. For several weeks she was unable to communicate verbally. When she was awake there were usually a lot of people in the room and so engagements tended to be very short. I did a little singing and then decided to risk dancing. My dancing is a fairly extreme therapy! I suggested that Alicia give her verdict by thumbs up, down or sideways. The first time I tried song and dance I was awarded a double thumbs down, but the cheeky smile suggested there was therapeutic engagement going on. Next time, a music therapist was playing a jig and so I did a very sketchy Morris-style dance, which was greeted with a double thumbs up. Although most of the follow-up to this has been song and conversation when it has become possible, my conclusion is that the dance and the humour that went with it enable a breakthrough in care that was therapeutic. The family always supported what I was doing. Alicia has made a lot of progress and is able to play with other children and go to different places in the hospital, including school, the play room and chapel. She was able to be a star in the nativity play in the carol service. I was overwhelmed when at the beginning of the service as I welcomed people, she came up to me and gave me an enormous hug.

Rev Nick Ball, chaplain

PRACTICE EXAMPLE 5.2: WORKING WITH A SIBLING

One example of creating a safe place is that of Josh (8), a sibling in the school who was in the hospital for a long period due to his brother's illness. Helping to design a tree, with blob shapes representing people, he chose different blobs for his family members and positioned them in ways that expressed aspects that were distinctive and special about each one. Sharing this creative task led to an outpouring of conversation about what it was like to spend long periods of time in hospital, and also the tremendous love and concern this young boy had for his family.

Rev Kathryn Darby, chaplain

Beginning the session well

Beginning the session well will involve an introduction and exchange of names, a clear explanation of potential activities, meeting the other family members, and gaining assent from the young people if they choose to do an activity. Showing young people the materials will give them a better indication of whether or not it is something they would like to participate in. There may be a need to 'warm up' to the exercise and to one another; for instance, making a bracelet with 3-year-old Zeb, the chaplain first just looked at the beads and talked about the colours and the ones that Zeb liked; then Zeb selected some beads that he liked and placed them in a bowl. One potential participant, Becky said 'no' to the initial invitation to take part, and then, seeing the materials, changed her mind. It may be most effective at times to show and demonstrate in order to help children consider the contact being offered and also to gauge their own readiness and confidence to take part.

Names are significant and it is important to determine what name is preferred by the young person: their full name, a shortened form or even a nickname. There are times when the hospital makes an error with recording names at the bed space, and on occasion parents have been reluctant to challenge mistakes! Within a multicultural setting names can signal culture, identity and a sense of belonging and are often a direct opportunity for getting to know a child better.

Ongoing consent

Voluntary informed consent should be an integral part of practice and children and young people should feel free to choose the level and extent to which they get involved. The spiritual care practitioner seeks to create a relaxed atmosphere and ensure that children know that any response is acceptable including choosing not to take part or continue. Seeking ongoing consent is an important part of maintaining a caring space. Being aware of body language and non-verbal cues, which may signal tiredness or the need to withdraw, are all elements of offering a safe space. Illness can bring particular vulnerabilities, and young people may be surprised themselves at their sudden drop in energy or ability to focus. Effective spiritual care develops a fine tuning of attitude and approach, adjusting the appropriate space given to a child in terms of the intensity of the contact, the physical space between the spiritual care practitioner and the child, the emotional space, the pace of the interaction and the length of time spent during a single visit. Making a return visit may often be something to offer, as rapport and trust is built up over a period of time. It is important to let young people know that they can always say, 'Not today, thank you' and to empower them to be the gatekeepers of their own space. On the other hand, sometimes a little gentle persuasion or showing them that a potential activity can raise their interest and help them to find new energy and a desire to engage can be an important part of recovery. Where a relationship truly develops with patients and often their family over time, there will be a degree of reciprocity. If an activity raises difficult issues for a child, then a referral could be made to the nurse in charge or other members of the multidisciplinary team.

Empowering children and young people to choose, ask, understand and express are all integral elements of best practice in spiritual care and give them agency in a context where there are few opportunities for this kind of self-assertion. It is important to respect the consent and will of the very young too; babies and toddlers will make it plain when they are happy or not with something. When young patients are given information and choice about participating in the activities in a hospital context this may lead them to value the conversation and interaction more.

Working in a containing way and ending well

Ending a session well is also important, particularly if a child or young person has been open about difficult feelings and experiences. Using spiritual care exercises can be highly engaging and revealing; working with tools has the potential to open the road quickly to less conscious material. There is a need also to work in a contained and containing way, valuing and acknowledging when precious insights have been shared by young people, giving reassurances and affirmation, and pacing the contact appropriately. One volunteer noted that 'working one-to-one for an hour with a child in the school seemed a long time to be working at depth and could be too intense'. Ending the session well will involve valuing the time spent with the individual or group of children, showing gratitude for their gifts shared, offering a prayer or blessing where appropriate to your role and the situation and explaining if and when there will be further contact.

Two chaplains, for instance, close the session of making bead bracelets by tying the strings for Eve (9) in hospital for spinal surgery and her sister, Maria (6), briefly reviewing what the beads represent, and thanking the girls for participating and noting Eve's courage. While the chaplain reflected later that the ending felt 'hasty', there is opportunity to revisit this encounter by visiting Eve again to talk about the bracelet and what was represented for her. It may be appropriate to leave something such as a visiting card, or postcard, with encouraging messages, prayers or readings as part of the farewell. Reflecting back on the session with the child can be a way to find appropriate closure. If time or interruption do not allow for a good ending, it might be possible to promise a return visit, with materials to build on a project, such as building a room for an elephant or reviewing the contents of a sensory box. Handover to other professionals, such as teachers, play specialists and youth workers or nurses might also be appropriate. Any concerns about mental health or safeguarding issues can be taken to the duty nurse or equivalent.

ACTIVITY 5.2: EXAMEN DOLL

The examen is a spiritual exercise associated with St Ignatius of Loyola. It is a way of reflecting on our feelings and state of being (see Appendix 2). It works well with children and young people across a wide age range. A child is invited to make a self-portrait on both sides of a stick figure with one side having a happy face and the other a sad face (wooden like a lolly stick readily available from craft suppliers), which can be easily accomplished using felt-tip pens. This simple prompt can help children to consider the happy and sad aspects in their life, what is strengthening as well as challenging, and all of this can be brought before God in a prayer, if appropriate, expressing what is difficult and asking for God's help, or noticing what has been uplifting in the day and offering gratitude. Katy (7) reflected on the things that made her happy: her new baby brother, her mum and her iPad – and things that made her sad – not being about to use the iPad, needles and snoring (a real issue when children have to sleep on the ward alongside adults!). Meeting with Daisy (8) on the oncology ward, we were aware that Daisy might have some anxiety and vulnerability about the fact that she was soon to receive a bone marrow transplant. There was also the ongoing issue of missing being with her family at home. While often bright and lively, Daisy was quiet and withdrawn. Making the examen doll and reflecting on this with us helped her to express some of her worries and concerns, as well as look for the sources of light and hope in her situation.

Rev Kathryn Darby and Rev Rachel Hill-Brown, chaplains

Moving deeper

Sometimes having fun on one occasion and building rapport in an easy and light-hearted way will lead to other times when deeper issues or concerns come to the surface. Introducing spiritual care activities can be a gentle way to offer non-threatening care and attention, without necessarily directly addressing core issues, particularly after experiencing trauma or sudden shock associated with illness or accidents. A shared activity can provide the focus and impetus of important conversation. Much as a mother cradles an infant, there are times, as children, young people and adults, when we need a holding space, a safe shelter, in order to find the comfort we need for wounds of the spirit to heal. Gradually, with gentle support, young people will find it is safe to entrust the difficult burdens, concerns and frustrations, as well as hopes and aspirations.

ACTIVITY 5.3: ISLAMIC BEAD BRACELETS

Zamir was visiting Sofia (9), who lived with a chronic condition and had been recently admitted when symptoms had become more acute. Introducing the beads activity (see Appendix 2), Zamir explained how the different coloured beads could represent different qualities and feelings, such as peace, courage, strength and love, or fear and sadness. The invitation was made to select those beads that represented what was important to Sofia. When exploring the theme of feeling safe, represented by the colour green, Sofia divulged her insecurities, describing how other children had made fun of her in the playground, her fear of being alone and bored at night and having to take medicine, though she knew it made her better.

Sofia wanted to have a bead of every colour on her bracelet and Zamir concluded to herself that Sofia may not have entirely understood her description of the exercise. However, when the bracelet was completed, Sofia explained the difference between the beads on her bracelet, pointing to two sections: 'These are the things that I already have, and these are the colours (and qualities) that I pray to Allah I will have.' For Sofia, this simple reflective exercise became a way of laying before Allah some of the deeper movements of her heart, her hopes and desires for her life.

It emerged that Sofia's mum played a major comforting and caring role, that the family prayed together and that prayer was very important in their journey with this illness. As they went through the beads they talked about how to ask God to make things better and how to thank God. Zamir suggested some prayers that Sofia could say at night and at those times when she felt scared, and they thought about all the wonderful things to be grateful for. Sofia was supported in exploring her world, and the presence and importance of her relationships with people and with God.

After the activity was finished, Sofia's mum spoke with Zamir about their plans for pilgrimage. They had taken an oath that they would perform the pilgrimage with Sofia if God made her well enough to travel without her oxygen. This had happened, and the family had plans for travelling in June. They spoke of their trust in God and how they felt that God had answered their prayers. Four days later, Zamir revisited Sofia who was wearing the bead bracelet. When asked how it made her feel, she said, 'Good!' and recounted what all the colours stood for, the fact that she wore it all the time except at night and that she had taken it off while she was cleaning her shoes, as she did not want it to get dirty. The bracelet continued to offer a reminder of the care of God and of the attention and care of the chaplain who visited her and promised to pray for her.

Zamir Hussain, chaplain

Fleeting encounters

Contact with a child or young person may be a one-off encounter or even a fleeting contact. We may only be able to create such space for a short time but it might be an important part of enabling a child or young person to make sense of their experience and gain some inner healing and resolution. Engaging in this kind of reflection while in the hospital context before returning to life at home and school, where friends often cannot identify with or particularly understand what their friend has experienced, can help a child or young person to leave some of the difficult memories and trauma behind and make a fuller recovery. Often this is more possible with a relative stranger.

ACTIVITY 5.4: SENSORY BOX

I spent time with Callum (16), who was due to be discharged that day. As a result of an accident, Callum had limited fine motor control and was still processing the shock of being involved in a road traffic accident. I offered a spiritual care activity of decorating a sensory box (Appendix 2). First, the young person is invited to decorate a medium-sized box, reflecting his or her unique personality. The box can then be filled with things that bring comfort, appealing to the five senses of taste, touch, hearing, smell and sight; for example, a small bar of chocolate, a soft toy, favourite music, a scented item, a photograph. While making the sensory box, Callum reflected with me about his accident, his hospital stay and the prospect of returning to sixth-form study.

Rev Kathryn Darby, chaplain

Working together

There can be advantages to working in twos. One spiritual care practitioner can engage with the parent or carer and free the other person to concentrate on an activity with the child or young person. This offers a different kind of space for all of the people concerned. Parents are given a rest from caring, and a chance to have an adult conversation and receive pastoral care while the young person is given freedom to explore independently. As an example of this, two chaplains approached Zara's family, one coming alongside Zara (13) with a tea light activity, while the other chaplain spent time talking with Zara's mother who was highly anxious and closely tied to the bedside. Offering this listening support helped to ease some of the fears, anxiety and isolation of Zara's mum, while Zara created something that brought smiles of enjoyment and a glow of pride to both of them. The atmosphere at the bedside was considerably different at the end of the pastoral encounter – Zara who had been listless and bored was animated and happy, and her mum looked more relaxed and comforted. A sense of confidence and trust had been built and a plan made for future contact. The effectiveness of the contact was the result of the parallel working. There are times, for instance, when a lone chaplain talking only to the parent can make matters more stressful for a child or young person who overhears the concerns of the parent.

PRACTICE EXAMPLE 5.3: ART ACTIVITIES WITH SONAM

Chaplaincy received a referral from the nurse manager to visit Sonam (15). Regular contact over a period of several months included work with glass paints, paper design, crafts and beads, and through this creative contact a mutual respect and understanding developed between Sonam and I. During her period of convalescence, which included highs and lows, stresses and challenges, as well as moments of achievement and connection with others, I discovered Sonam's artistic talent, and other staff admired the pillow case that Sonam decorated elaborately with flowers, intricate lines and colours using fabric pens. One day, at my request, Sonam decorated my hand with a mendi design. We were both able to grow in awareness and understanding of each other's faith background – Christianity and Hinduism – and share simple prayers of blessing on occasion. As the date for discharge approached, Sonam prepared gifts and cards to thank staff for their care and support. I was very touched by the beautifully decorated burlap bag that she gave me, and the message of thanks:

> Thank you so much for all your support and all of your help. I loved doing all the fun, arty things you brought with you. You helped me through my journey even at the most difficult times. I will always remember your kindness and soft words of hope, encouragement and love. Thank you! Love, Sonam

(P.S. Hope you like this)

> On the reverse side of the card was a colourful design resembling the mendi art that we had shared, a special and valued memento of an important relationship within the hospital and a shared journey.
>
> *Rev Kathryn Darby, chaplain*

Simple gifts and kindnesses

We can offer one another the most simple and yet profound gift that we have: the gift of our presence. One of the chaplaincy volunteers, now retired, recalled an early experience of a hospital admission which lasted many weeks. This period in her life had been extremely difficult, at a time when hospital visiting for parents was much more restricted, and she had felt frightened and confused. She remembers the visits from the hospital chaplain who brought a cheerful reassuring presence and she remembers the small gift that he brought for her which was not particularly costly or rare. And yet, while most of the memories of that time are hazy and blurred, the kindness of the chaplain and his small gift is the thing that she vividly recalls.

Sometimes kindness is expressed in unexpected ways. One of our Roman Catholic chaplains, Sister Thérèse, was in the bookshop at St Chad's Cathedral in Birmingham and was buying several copies of *My Hospital Prayer and Activities Book* (Scott 2013), one of the few resources written specifically for hospitalised children. One of the customers enquired about the books she was holding and Sister Thérèse explained they were for the children at the hospital over the road, and that person then offered to buy all ten books! These books are given out to our Roman Catholic patients. Having told this story to various people, others are now fundraising to provide the books for our patients.

ACTIVITY 5.5: SPIRITUAL CARE BLANKETS

A volunteer called Anne makes small quilts for the chaplaincy department, which feature different shapes, pictures, animals, emblems, colours, patterns and colourful fabrics. A blanket can be specially selected for children or young people based on their own particular story. One child liked butterflies and this image of new life and transformation was given to her as a picture of hope and comfort during a difficult time on the intensive care ward. On one occasion, a 5-year-old girl was feeling upset after a major heart operation and offering a blanket became both a comfort and a distraction. Another child who had struggled with an intense period of illness was offered a quilt with a puppy dog pattern to link with the positive, recent experience of having a visit from his beloved dog at the hospital.

Malgosia (4) was in hospital recovering from a liver transplant. She was in the PICU, and her mother was alongside her. Although she had a few words of English, her first language was Romanian, and her mother struggled to express even a few words in English. Malgosia appeared to be drifting in and out of sleep as a colleague and I came alongside them both at the bedside, the doctors discussing her case at the foot of her bed. After pointing to different blankets on Malgosia's bed to define the word 'blanket', I asked the mother if she would like one of the special quilts from chaplaincy as a gift for Malgosia, and offered a blanket with a pretty butterfly pattern. Malgosia's face lit up with a smile as it was presented to her. I was surprised at how conscious she evidently was and by the strength of her response. 'She likes animals', her mother explained, and I was pleased that this match had been made with Malgosia's own interests. My colleague and I admired the animals already on her bed, moving them and interacting with her as we made her teddies dance and play. We shared in a short blessing and said farewell.

Rev Kathryn Darby, chaplain and Hayley Painter, spiritual care volunteer

Protecting privacy

Although creating space for encounters and relationships is a priority for spiritual care, we need to hold this in tension with a need for privacy in a setting where many people may invade space, ask questions and require a response at a time when a child may not want to give one.

Engaging with children at their bedside can be a particularly intimate encounter, and spiritual care practitioners observe that sensitive discernment is required in cultivating safe spaces. A chaplain's visit may be interrupted by those attending to the child's medical needs; this needs to be managed effectively in order to safeguard the child's sense of privacy. As chaplains become more integrated into the multidisciplinary team, it can be best practice to schedule in sessions with the family, in the way of physiotherapists, psychologists and consultants or any other professional. While chaplains will often 'loiter with intent', there is also room for working more strategically, setting up appointments for spiritual care sessions, and communicating with the wider professional team about intentions and observations.

Holy ground

Designated religious spaces can provide a sacred space distinct from the surrounding medical environment in which to mark a significant stage in the child's spiritual journey, such as transition from hospital to home, or recognising grief or loss (e.g. lighting a candle or making a prayer for the prayer tree for a friend who has died). On the other hand, it may be that more neutral spaces without connection to religious culture or tradition provide the more likely environment for sacred connections, particularly for people who are living on the margins of, or outside, faith traditions.

Celebrating festivals can be a dimension of spiritual care which has a religious element. For example, chaplains took materials to the mental health ward to celebrate the Buddhist festival of Wesak, marking the birth and enlightenment of Buddha. A few simple materials helped to create an inviting space for the children and young people to enter: some green and shimmering blue pieces of fabric draped on the floor to create the image of a river, some scattered flower petals, a bowl of rhododendrons, some peaceful music, dimmed lights. The young people came into a tranquil and inviting space and sat down with enjoyment and some amusement with the chaplains on the floor. They shared in a half hour of reflection, mindfulness and simply being together in the comforting space, while exploring the practices of one of the world's religions. Sometimes, simple approaches are the best means of offering spiritual care. In working with young people with depression, the leader may be looking for ways to change the energy in the room, and changing the focus can help to do this, for instance, inviting people to sit on the floor, as in the Wesak example, or sharing in an activity. For celebrating

Diwali, the chaplains brought candle holders to paint, Indian sweets, colouring sheets and simple information about the festival to the ward. However, it is always important to ask staff about bringing food.

PRACTICE EXAMPLE 5.4: LAUREN'S CANDLE HOLDER

Liz visited Lauren with spiritual care activities over a period of weeks. While designated 'Church of England', nothing had been said about organised religion by Lauren's parents, although Liz spoke at times about the love and care of God in relation to activities shared. Near the end of the weeks of treatment, Liz gave Lauren a candle holder to decorate and a battery-operated light to keep within it, talking about how sometimes people light candles for prayers. This sparked a conversation about the fact that Lauren's dad had once been an altar boy and had been confirmed. After weeks of listening and spending time together, matters of faith and religious tradition were raised. Lauren said she would like to put her new candle holder in her special 'God shelter', a playhouse in the garden that she shared with her sister. While not a child who often attended church, Lauren had ideas about God and a special God place at home.

Liz Bryson, spiritual care volunteer

Creating a safe distance

There are ways to listen to the child's story indirectly. A spiritual care practitioner may get into a conversation with the child's toys and teddies on their bed in order to engage with the child who will project their feelings and views onto the toy. Often, these toys are highly significant, having travelled with the child through various stages of illness, been with them during operations, or represent the love and care of family members. Relating to a teddy also allows the child to observe and decide if the spiritual care practitioner is trustworthy in their attitudes and approach. Sam (2) was somewhat wary of the chaplain initially, wondering perhaps if she was another adult about to perform another test, injection or necessary prodding. But the chaplain made it plain that she was only interested in a time of light-hearted fun with a hand puppet she had brought in her bag and blowing bubbles. Soon Sam was joining in with the animation, smiling and laughing and getting to know the chaplain and the puppet. At the end of the visit, Sam took

'Mousy' the puppet and kissed his nose with real affection. Expressing and receiving love in safe ways provides a good tonic for the spirit.

Reflecting on things such as how one demonstrates love and care, including touch where appropriate, and the importance of smiling and shared non-verbal communication are all essential elements in judging the distance appropriately between adult and child.

PRACTICE EXAMPLE 5.5: DANI'S FACES

Dani was a 4-year-old who had been undergoing treatment for cancer. She had developed an infection which lead to a respiratory arrest and a cardiac arrest. This meant a long spell in intensive care and a long recovery process. Dani went from a bright chatty little girl to a child who could hardly hold up her own head. Dani was receiving a list of support from physiotherapy, occupational therapy and speech and language therapy but had not yet recovered her speech. I knew her family well and had spent lots of time with Dani doing a range of activities and supporting her and her family. Dani appeared happy in herself, but her limited ability to communicate meant that we were not entirely sure she was happy. So using stickers with facial expressions, I worked with Dani to help her make a card (which I designed to fit in the communication folder given to her by her speech and language therapist). Using the facial expressions and assigning them to feelings (happy, sad, worried, excited, hurting) Dani was able to look at and, in time, point to the face which showed how she felt. We used it to play games with, but also as a serious tool to help her express how she was feeling. She liked it and her mum found it a reassuring tool to use on quite a regular basis.

In terms of spiritual care, this activity helped Dani to express herself in challenging circumstances. It also gave her some control and promoted her self-confidence and self-esteem. It brought her a sense of contentment and reassurance. It helped her to make meaning and connections and to communicate these with others. Dani recovered fairly quickly and was able to start talking again within a few weeks. But some months later she still had the card to hand and her mum described how it had become quite a treasured possession. Dani simply described it as 'important when I was poorly'.

Rev Rachel Hill-Brown, chaplain

Empowerment

There are situations and conditions which leave children and young people even more disempowered than usual, for instance, if held in any kind of traction or attached to a ventilator or unable to move from the bed for any number of reasons.

When children are particularly vulnerable

We need to be sure that we are not opening up areas that are overly sensitive when children and young people are particularly vulnerable, for instance when they are spending time on the intensive care unit or are recovering from recent operations. It is important to be vigilant in assessing energy levels, giving opportunity for children to continue a project on another day. On the other hand, strength can be gained through spiritual care activities at critical times. Janey (12) had been admitted onto the PICU and was struggling with her breathing, the effects of a severe asthma attack, and her sense of panic was making the situation worse. Sensing her anxiety, the parents were also becoming increasingly upset and this in turn may have been causing Janey's anxiety to escalate. Using beads to make a bracelet with Janey, the chaplain helped her to relax, drawing her attention away from her anxiety and focusing on the simple exercise, taking pleasure in making something beautiful and getting to know a friendly face in an unfamiliar and perhaps frightening environment. At the same time her parents were given the opportunity to take a few minutes' break in the family room.

Pet therapy

Sometimes spiritual care activities will highlight the importance of pets to children. Pets often feature in family illustrations, and are mentioned in prayers. Recently, on the PICU, a child who was in palliative care was united with his pet dog on the unit. Offering a blanket to that child with a dog pattern was a way of providing further care and appreciation of this child's identity in relation to his pet. Another child, Annie (13), who was fairly non-communicative, and generally low in mood, was transformed when her beloved pet was brought onto the ward. Staff concerned about Annie's dispiritedness had recognised the importance of her relationship with her dog through her many pictures, and as a result organised this important piece of spiritual care. Children and young people will enjoy telling stories of their pets or sharing pictures with others.

ACTIVITY 5.6: EASTER CHICKS

In helping to plan an Easter visit, Alice asked, 'Can you bring live chicks? That would make my Easter!' When the Hindu and Christian chaplains arrived for their Celebrate visit (see page 130), Alice shot into the room, and asked, 'Have you got the chicks?!' It is essential to be reliable when relating to young people with mental health difficulties who may have suffered disappointments, hurts and loss, especially in their early life.

We started the session with decorating biscuits and chocolate eggs and gradually others peeped their heads around the door and joined the party. Offering a non-compulsory session is distinct from other scheduled contact with teachers, therapists and psychologists – a space that people can choose to enter that holds a relaxed and undemanding feel about it, in an environment where choice is limited. The atmosphere was relaxed and easygoing with decorating and eating biscuits and chocolates, and making paper chains, sharing conversation with a couple of the nurses joining in, and a little face painting: a chick painted on a cheek. Even though it is a small thing to paint a chick on someone's face, there is care and also touch, while a quiet stillness and opportunity to talk can also develop. Then the nurse announced, 'They're here!' – and soon the young people each had a chick in their hand, cooing and sighing over them, expressing wonder and delight and taking turns holding them.

Chicks have an appeal because they are soft, non-threatening and vulnerable; there are lessons to be learned from them about our own attitude and approach to children and young people when seeking to communicate acceptance and love. Josie exclaimed suddenly, as we were returning the chicks to their box, 'Thanks – I love the chaplains' visit! This is the best one yet!' Her spontaneous remark was golden. Creating spaces where compassion is given and received is the heart and soul work of chaplaincy. The expression of unconditional love brings meaningful connection. Rakesh reflected, 'We don't need to say a lot, this is not a platform for a didactic approach, but an opportunity to create spaces for the children to experience something positive and to build relationships of trust.'

Visiting the eating disorders ward, rather than biscuits, we gave out little tiny decorative chicks, carefully placing the little pieces of fluff into the hands of children, nurses and a couple of visiting parents, who all received these tiny gifts with pleasure and thanks. We also brought out Easter paper chains and they enjoyed this small gift. It's often the small things that communicate kindness, that are invested with meaning and transformed by the connections made between people. Leaving an ornamental chick behind might reawaken for some the memory of holding the chicks and the positive experience of simply being together in the warmth of that moment in the shelter of a safe and caring group.

Rakesh Bhatt and Rev Kathryn Darby, chaplains

Recognising the spiritual resources of children and young people

Often in a hospital the focus is on the illness and helping a child or young person to get better. They become the focus of received care. And yet, it is vital to recognise that children and young people have a spiritual dimension and resources which are already present and which will become evident and which they may wish to share. For instance, they bring a sense of play, imagination, honesty, reflective and open-hearted searching and questioning, trust, wisdom through experience, care giving and sensitivity to others. Creating spaces for such spiritual gifts to emerge and be celebrated is an essential part of a movement towards healing, growth and wholeness. The spiritual care practitioner too will go away changed by the encounter, encouraged in their own spirituality.

ACTIVITY 5.7: DREAM SPACE

Dream Space was a project developed with the play and youth work department of the hospital and designed to give children and young people the opportunity to decorate an art canvas (A4 size) using paints, stickers, felt pens, fabric, patterned paper, buttons and decorative pieces in order to portray a 'dream space' through collage, colour, pattern and texture: a favourite place, imagined or real, to express their hopes and dreams. The purpose of the project was to encourage them to think beyond the moment and to dream.

For some, this might have felt more risky than for others, but by affirming individuality, self-expression and creativity the hope was to see them make connections and meaning through using imagination. Giving children and young people space to express these dreams and listening to their stories is an important way of nurturing and supporting them.

The strengths of Dream Space are many: it is accessible for both spiritual care practitioners and young people and it is versatile, adaptable, wide ranging, suitable for children of all ages, ability, and both genders; lends itself to working at depth and provides scope for further reflection; it is fun to engage in and leads to very pleasing results after relatively little time and effort if children and young people are very poorly or limited in their ability. Some of the main themes emerging were: being together with family, being well; holiday dream locations; the importance of home; hopes, aspirations and struggles; overcoming adversity; and it expressed the complexity of dealing with sickness. The pictures were gathered together to form a display in the chapel, giving opportunity for the children to take pride and enjoyment in their work.

Charlotte Frith, youth worker and Rev Rachel Hill-Brown, chaplain

Summary

Creating positive spaces for spiritual care involves awareness of self and others and the physical and emotional space between. Core good practice elements include:

- Being non-judgemental, listening, accepting, affirming and being attentive.

- Beginning and ending a session well offers an appropriate holding space.

- Gaining ongoing voluntary informed consent.

- Using activities to help build rapport and open the way to deeper conversations.

- Chapels or other religious rooms can provide an appropriate space for religious and spiritual care, particularly at times of transition, but more neutral spaces can also become the ground in which the sacred is noticed or shared.

Chapter 6

Meaning Making with Children and Young People

PRACTICE EXAMPLE 6.1: PETER AND DIANA'S PICTURES

The youth worker was doing the Dream Space activity with some young people on the mental health unit. While one young person, Peter, worked silently during the creative session, his picture was revealing in the words he chose to paint: to have hope; to have freedom; to have goals; to have motivation. On the accompanying tag and description of the picture he wrote, 'It is where I want to be and what I want to have in the future after I am treated.' The nursing staff were pleased to gain understanding about this young person who was suffering with depression and had not been able to articulate much about his experience.

Diana used the Dream Space opportunity to describe a near death experience when she felt drawn by a warm and inviting light that offered peace and rest and the inner struggle and commitment which led her back to consciousness. Words on the borders of her picture indicated important themes in her life, 'To walk on my own/ Knowing I'm never far from home'; 'Come walk beside me'; 'You're my shining star' and symbols: a black background, an inner ball of light, a purple person and hearts. Offering a variety of materials – stickers, words, paints, fabric, and patterned paper – enabled a depth of expression and exploration of meaning.

Kim Caves, youth worker

Facilitating meaning making is an integral part of spiritual care and it may be that illness leads to questions that need exploring for children and young people and their families. It is in exploring meaning making that religious care may also become part of what is being offered, and for some young people and their families meaning making needs to be done in relation to their faith as well.

PRACTICE EXAMPLE 6.2: DILAN'S STORY (PART 1)

For some, an act of spiritual care will have more meaning, depth and richness if it is an act of religious care. There may be ways to take the images and symbols which are already important, such as seahorses, birds or other animals, hearts and precious objects and find their link into the religious narrative. Dilan (8) had been treated for several weeks on the intensive care ward for an infection that had left him paralysed and in shock. The critical point had been passed, and he was making a slow recovery. Dilan belonged to a Christian family for whom prayer and faith were immensely important; he liked to sing in church and enjoyed stories and church life. The book *Josh Stays in Hospital* was a good gift to offer, a Christian story about another little boy who looked about 9 years old and had to stay in hospital over Christmas. His mum said that Dilan had had some disturbing dreams, and this had evoked some fears in him about the family being all together. There was some processing to do – healing of his spirit – and he needed support in making sense of all that had happened in his life, the separation he had experienced and fears he had suffered while going through this health crisis.

I asked Dilan, 'Do you want to continue the story?' 'Yes', he nodded. We read the story, and I asked him, 'Do you remember the story of Jesus who is in the boat with the disciples, and stills the storm?' Dilan remembered that story and we reflected a little on the story together. We also read how Josh, a character in the story, makes a prayer for the prayer tree – a sad and a happy face on the star prayers. After the story we made a prayer leaf for Dilan, with a stamp picture of two butterflies and love hearts; I wrote the names of each person in the family on the leaf as Dilan spelled out the name of his brother and told me how to spell his name. I talked about the meaning of a butterfly emerging from a cocoon, like Dilan finding his voice and emerging with new strength from his illness – how his voice was already so much stronger, and each day he was getting much better. We talked about the picture of the hearts representing the love of the family, each for the other one. We made two leaves, with the butterflies, the hearts and the names of Joe and his family: one for his bed space, and one for him to put on the prayer tree later, with his dad and mum. Some weeks later, Dilan referred to this activity and the prayer leaf that we prepared in detail. It is an example of meaning making drawing on faith, story and action.

Rev Kathryn Darby, chaplain

Using metaphor

Metaphors are a way of exploring meaning and they can help children and young people explore their spiritual needs. When linked with their hospital experience, metaphors have the potential to go on nurturing them, long after they have left the hospital, reminding them of what they have overcome, helping them to cling to the light in the midst of change and ongoing recovery. Metaphors can be explored in many ways including through stories, artefacts, toys, art and activities and there are times when they open up a new language for exploring spirituality. They are equally useful with families as with children. They may also be useful for work with staff. Fruitfulness as an alternative to success, for example, may be a helpful way of reflecting on spiritual care (Nash 2014).

ACTIVITY 6.1: STONE PAINTING

Visiting Eleana on the day before a major operation, I drew a bunny on one side of the stone, and the 3-year-old helped to choose colours to decorate this stone (to go in an Easter garden). Asking Eleana's mum what message might be included on the reverse side, she suggested, 'Bounce back', reflecting the very real story of her own daughter who had endured many operations and interventions and had managed to bounce back in astonishing ways. The following day, Eleana was in the theatre for many hours, and it was an agonising wait for her family. Spending some time in the chapel, Eleana's mum noticed the garden and the small pathway built from stones decorated by the children. Her eye landed on the stone that Eleana had helped to make the day before and the message, 'Bounce back', which gave hope, inspiration and consolation.

Rev Kathryn Darby, chaplain

Some of the metaphors that we have found helpful include butterflies, rainbow, lion, swan paddling hard underneath but gliding on the surface, hospital as prison or bubble, riding an emotional roller coaster, writing a book page by page not knowing what comes next, getting stuck, parallel universe, iceberg. We hear these and other metaphors from young people and their families, as well as introducing them ourselves. Research with nurses suggests that 'the creative use of language, phrases and metaphors may also support nurses to talk about difficult topics and so reduce the likelihood of defensive or blocking behaviours during times of stress and anxiety' (Appleton and Flynn 2014, p.382).

PRACTICE EXAMPLE 6.3: WE ARE DIAMONDS

I spent some time with Ria yesterday and she said something really beautiful. We were talking about the TV series, *Children's Hospital: The Chaplains*, and she told me how gorgeous Wilf was, and her nan said he must have been a favourite (see Practice Examples 7.4 and 8.7). I said, 'We are not allowed to have favourites.' Ria grinned and said, 'The thing is, we are all like diamonds – special, individual and unique. But you get to spend more time with some of us than others and then you get to see how beautiful we really are.'

Rev Rachel Hill-Brown, chaplain

There are issues to consider in using metaphor. Some may be culturally or personality specific and can be part of a coping strategy or a powerful hook to hold on to during the treatment journey. What works for one child and family may not necessarily work for another in a similar situation; they are very individual. Nevertheless, there is evidence to suggest that peer explanations can be helpful in learning how to talk about illness (Whaley 1994, p.202). Metaphors do not always work, however, and we need to consider developmental issues and capacity to understand and process such language. Thus, Eric has Asperger's syndrome and also a complex physical condition that required frequent operations and hospital admissions. Showing him the picture of St Christopher carrying Christ over the fast-flowing river of life, as an illustration of how people in the community were praying for Eric and 'carrying him through' his current situation, took some unpacking! 'But I am not being carried by Christopher,' he said, looking puzzled. However, offering Eric a fabric gold heart for every member of his family to glue onto the card, including his grandparents, his two dogs, and his immediate family – amounting to 12 hearts – did prove to be a satisfying activity that included some metaphor and provided him with a creative focus for prayer. He decided to keep his new card under his pillow.

ACTIVITY 6.2: CHESS AS A METAPHOR FOR DYING

We can use metaphors with patients and their families to explore issues. The game of chess is a powerful and multifaceted metaphor for the struggle against mortality and is one which resonates with some children, young people and their families. Chess is a battle between two forces; it basically has three stages: the opening, the middle game and the endgame. The opening can be likened to the diagnostic stage – what is your opponent's plan? In the middle game, the forces of medicine, character, love and prayer fight against the illness. Sometimes the opponent threatens in more than one way. Complex illnesses are more difficult to fight. A move that attacks one part of the opposition can leave you weaker to fend off other attacks. In the analogy the endgame begins when we know that the opponent is being defeated (i.e. no longer a threat to life or wellbeing) or when we recognise that the illness is terminal and life is limited. In the latter case, we do not know how long the endgame will go on, but we do know that even the best moves we make will not be enough to defeat the illness. In the endgame we have a choice between playing defensively to prolong life as long as possible or we can play a more risky game, in which quality of life, probably expressed in fulfilling as many bucket list wishes as possible, is the main objective. Either way, an Advance Care Plan can enable discussions about a good death and funeral. The game can end with dignity and peace and a sense that though we have lost, we have done our best and found real consolation. The different pieces can also represent different aspects of the struggle, but the main point is the thought-out battle to save life.

Rev Nick Ball, chaplain

Art

Artwork can be a way of exploring metaphor and engaging with mystery and the depths of human experience and spirituality. In an exceptional illustration of this, the artwork of Katie Bryson was shared at BCH.

Katie designed pottery shapes that could sit comfortably in an adult hand, a sphere, but not perfectly formed, rather holding blemishes and bumps, rough patches and smooth, representing the way that life leaves us scarred and bruised at times. At the top of the sphere is a hole that one can peek through into the inside of the pottery piece and view the darker interior, also containing colour and beauty. The inside of the sphere, which can be viewed, but holds some mystery too, represents the inner life of the person that is precious and central, formed within, even in the midst of life's challenges and trials. Katie made many of these exquisite clay pieces which were brought in to the chaplaincy by her mother and became special gifts that could be shared with others. Katie's own story was one of immense faith amidst suffering; diagnosed with cancer at 10 years, she lived until she was 27. Art was both her gift and expressive means of telling her story and engaging with her circumstances. Her delicate and inspiring pieces of art brought hope, inspiration and beauty to individuals who were invited to consider that while 'stuff happens' and our outer appearance may show signs of the struggle we have endured, within ourselves, our beautiful and unique identity is being formed and the whole of us (represented in this pottery which was lovely to look at and to hold) is wondrous. The fact that this art came from Katie and was born out of her own struggle, faith and vision was an especially poignant and powerful example of the scope of metaphor.

ACTIVITY 6.3: BLOB PICTURES

Blob Pictures (see www.pipwilson.com) come in a range of configurations and contexts, suitable for making an initial contact with a child or young person. At a glance, children can indicate who they identify with in the Blob Picture and a genuine child-centred conversation can begin. Lou met Thomas for the first time and invited him to pick the blob figure that was like him in some way and suggested that he might like to draw a face on it that showed how he was feeling. Thomas said that he felt angry sometimes, and proceeded to talk about his sisters, family relationships, his feelings about the hospital school, which he liked, and missing his friends.

Lou Langford, spiritual care volunteer

Asking open-ended questions about pictures and artwork
When looking at pictures with children, it is important to ask open-ended questions such as 'Tell me about your picture', 'What is happening here in the picture?', 'What is this about?' or 'How does the person feel inside this picture?' If appropriate, you might ask, 'What do you think this person would want to say to God about what has happened in the story?' Avoid making assumptions about the pictures children and young people have made. Chaplains are not psychologists but can be listeners of dreams and can ask questions that open the conversation up, resisting analysis and drawing conclusions. They can also listen well and create spaces so that a child or young person may reveal something of their inner life.

Taking artworks and tangible objects home, such as postcards or bracelets, that connect with their experience may become symbols that remind the child of their important time in hospital and help them to integrate both the good and the bad from that experience.

ACTIVITY 6.4: ELEPHANT IN THE ROOM
Together with the play and youth work department, chaplaincy developed a project called The Elephant in the Room (Appendix 2) as a way of creating space to express the unspoken or difficult aspects of a child or young person's experience. In families, there is often an element of protecting one another from pain and suffering, and a conspiracy of silence develops. However, not talking about areas of tension and concern can further complicate matters. Drawing from the meaning of the poem, 'The Elephant in the Room' (www.irisremembers.com/poemsandstories/viewPoem.cfm?poemID=63) which describes the experience of people avoiding talking about the pain of grief, we designed an activity using decopatch and elephant figures as a potential platform for discussing what might be difficult or even considered taboo to say. One of the most fascinating encounters was with a young person who created a yellow elephant to go in a yellow room because nobody saw her problems. Rachel, the chaplain, met with Anna (16) who was receiving treatment for a brain tumour. Anna had recently had surgery through her nose and was preparing to go home.

As materials for the Elephant in the Room were set out, Anna's dad took the opportunity to go out for some fresh air. Parents can benefit

---

indirectly by gaining a little private recovery space for themselves away from the bedside when their child is secure and engaged with a chaplain. Anna was well aware of the Elephant in the Room poem: 'I know all about that, we did it in English last year.' She talked confidently about her illness and treatment and the impact it was having on her and her family. In discussion about the elephant and meaning, Anna talked about the way that her younger siblings did not talk to her about her illness; she sensed that they worry but did not know how to respond to them. She also described the openness with her own parents in talking about her condition and concluded that, for them, the elephant was more about not wanting to see one another upset or tearful. As her dad returned, she immediately stopped talking. In this instance, it would have been helpful to have a follow-up visit to pursue the conversation, but in itself, the seeds for further reflection and possibly new ways of communicating had been planted.

Another simpler version of the Elephant in the Room is to take an elephant picture that children can colour and use as a focus for reflection. Working with Charlotte (14) in this way, the chaplain had a long conversation about life in general, about Charlotte's faith in God and how she felt being in hospital. While colouring, Charlotte wrote significant words on her elephant picture – scared, God, family – which led to a more directed and increasingly prayerful conversation.

Rev Rachel Hill-Brown, chaplain

Taking care of objects made

Children and young people take pride in their work and may surprise themselves with what they are able to achieve. Some of the objects, such as the elephants covered in decopatch, the decorated sensory boxes and the Dream Space pictures were particularly beautiful. We have also learnt that our intention for objects might not be what transpires for the young person. For example, we were using the Elephant in the Room metaphor to explore difficult and hidden feelings and issues and this sometimes contrasted sharply with the beautiful objects which resulted from the activity.

Appreciating and admiring objects made and sharing in the creative journey will help build self-esteem, self-confidence and resilience for children and young people who in their physical frailty may be struggling to maintain strength of spirit. Children often want to have their photograph taken with their pieces of work, or, if they were being displayed, assured of their safekeeping and made aware of how they could view these displays. In an uncertain and changing environment it is vital to communicate clearly and offer safety and security for any precious objects made. When introducing activities, the spiritual care practitioner must be clear about what will happen to the pieces that are made if they are to be part of a shared project for future display. Handling these objects and displaying them needs to be done with care. Often, through the process of making something in the company of a caring, attentive adult, objects become representative of significant discoveries and meaning for the young people, who may have travelled some distance in the session, both in their level of sharing and in the meaning invested in the exercise. They may have formed an attachment to both the object and to the person who has related to them. While agreeing to contribute to a common display at the beginning of the exercise, they may decide they want to take their picture home, and we must be flexible. One child wished to store his precious artwork in a 'glass box'. His piece, along with the artwork of other children, was placed in a glass display cabinet in a hospital corridor for wider appreciation. Offering display opportunities can build self-esteem and a sense of belonging and community spirit.

PRACTICE EXAMPLE 6.4: BEN'S LANTERN

It may surprise us to discover the depth of meaning that has become associated with objects made in hospital when stress and insecurity are heightened. One example was visiting Ben during the palliative stage of his illness. His advancing brain tumour had led to some paralysis and lack of mobility and fine motor skills, but he was game to make a Chinese lantern as part of a festival celebration. I was touched to find this lantern hanging on his medical equipment by his bedside at home shortly before he died. He had bothered to bring it with him on his last trip out of hospital. My time spent with Ben had been precious, and I had always left my encounters with him lifted and encouraged by Ben's infectious humour, stories, optimism and vitality of spirit. He, in turn, gave me a religious medallion. Concrete reminders, objects made and exchanged, of the invisible bonds of love and care shared at the most tender of times in life are irreplaceable.

Rev Kathryn Darby, chaplain

Connecting

While they may be supported by family and friends, children or young people are in some ways alone with their illness and, therefore, building community is vital. It is important to acknowledge that spiritual needs and patient engagement with spirituality exist and continue, and that we just see glimpses of it. Sometimes, it is the things that we say and do, almost unaware, that will be the elements of lasting spiritual care.

Often, beginning a spiritual care activity with one child will create opportunities to include others and to build community within the hospital. This can also lead to shared meaning making. For example, a spiritual care practitioner visited a 9-year-old boy called Jamie with a cardboard tube, tissue paper, pens and stickers to make a viewfinder. Soon, a neighbouring child became involved and made one too. The viewfinder was used to notice things in the hospital that we might be thankful for, and to write these on the decorated tube. Both children enjoyed their time together and wrote the names of each other on their new viewfinders. Similarly, approaching one 6-year-old girl (recovering from a neck injury) with magic clay and bubbles became appealing for the older girl across the aisle, who came to join in the activity and to share a happy time together. Through the contact around the activity, the girls were able to share things with one another about why they were in the hospital, what they enjoyed, the recent film they had both seen and some of their favourite characters. The siblings of another small child arrived to visit their sister and appeared uncertain and insecure in the strange hospital environment. Soon they were also joining in with the activities. The activities provided by chaplaincy provided a platform for children to meet, be put at ease and become friends.

ACTIVITY 6.5: SAFE SPACE

One staff member involved young people in imagining a safe space and using clay to represent their safe/peaceful space. One person remembered a happy space with friends, where she had a strong sense of belonging, adventure and enjoyment of nature. This memory and image, symbolised in the clay model, was a sustaining image through difficult times. The group experience itself had offered a safe space for the young people. Working alongside them and making her own clay model, the staff member engaged with the young people in a gentle and non-confrontational way.

Tamsin Cuthbert, children's worker

Profound spiritual conversations

After a few visits made with spiritual care activities, children and young people may come to expect some kind of activity to be included in a visit, particularly if they are long-stay patients. Ria (Practice Example 6.3, Activity 6.6), for instance, will ask: 'What have you got for me today?' or 'I'm on the phone right now but could you come back in a few minutes with an activity please?' Spiritual care activities can be offered in openness to what may or may not emerge. There is a sense of spontaneity when carrying a number of activity options and being prepared to make something up on the spot. The intentionality comes in the attitude, the openness, the relational depth, the spiritual/faith awareness of the spiritual care practitioner. When we become involved in making something together, Ria often speaks profoundly about life and her observations about human behaviour and how it is, revealing high levels of patience, tolerance and acceptance about a situation that she cannot change but must endure at times: long spells in hospital, inconclusive procedures, waiting and wondering what next.

Through all of this, however, I believe that Ria has a highly developed spiritual awareness and sensitivity. For instance, when making a simple picture one day, I described the chapel to Ria. She commented, 'The chapel must be very important to some people, to go into when their child is in the hospital. Just to have a quiet place where they can go and sit and find some peace. Not that it can all be made better, but they can find some relief, some comfort. It doesn't make it all better, but it helps ease their pain. I understand about this,' she said, 'because after my grandpa died, my gran often went into the garden for some quiet and peace, and it helps her.' Ria also spoke of how she likes to have times of quiet when she can reflect privately.

Flow of conversation and communication

In their encounters with children and young people, spiritual care practitioners describe a flow of conversation and a depth of contact and communication, when the young person begins to take the lead. One chaplain, Lou Langford, describes her time with Jameel, 'There was an ease about this encounter; that is, I wasn't working hard to facilitate a conversation. While Jameel was engaged in the ordinary activity of colouring I was trusted with a flow of his thoughts and feelings. At such times I feel that I inhabit holy ground.' When a conversation or contact finds this kind of energy, directed by the child and entrusted to an adult, there can be the sense of being on the edge of something deeper, something difficult to articulate, but real. Such moments can carry immense meaning and sacredness, helping to establish a relationship of trust between the chaplain and the young people and their families. Such experiences are likely to flow when an activity brings a creative focus into the frame.

ACTIVITY 6.6: DECORATING A TEA LIGHT HOLDER

Glass tea light holders are simple and cheap to buy and can be decorated with appropriate pens and adapted to a range of contexts and purposes, such as Mother's day, Christmas, birthdays, etc. Ria described how, on a Saturday evening, the family loves to get together in the lounge – and they light lots of tea lights and candles and have a chill-out time together when listening to music and talking about the week and what has been going on. 'Because everyone is busy in the week with work and school, we have this lovely time together when we can catch up with what is going on with each other.' It was such a beautiful awareness that she had of the importance of being together in peaceful candlelit environment, sharing the events and feelings of the week.

Rev Kathryn Darby, chaplain

PRACTICE EXAMPLE 6.5: WORKING WITH HOLLY

Sometimes verbal communication is difficult because of developmental or illness issues. Maddy visited Holly, who was 14, but clearly had a much lower mental age and was largely non-verbal with only three or four words in her vocabulary including 'Daddy' and 'Mummy'. Maddy laid out three activities for Holly to choose from. When shown the scratch art wristband, which could be tailor-made and wrapped around the wrist for comfort, Holly showed great glee and enthusiasm and the activity was started. Maddy showed Holly her example wristband with a rainbow, a heart and a star already drawn and, in turn, Holly nodded that she would like these images on her wristband, along with her name. Her fine motor skills and strength were limited, but Maddy assisted her in making her design.

Next, Maddy suggested a stick person, drawing a happy and sad side, the Examen Doll activity. When they came to colouring in the stick person, Holly pointed to the rainbow and indicated that she wanted to make a rainbow on the sad side of her stick person. Maddy talked about the significance of the rainbow and how the rain comes first, but is followed by a rainbow, just as a rainy day may be followed by a brighter day. Mum interjected at this point, 'She certainly had a grumpy day yesterday!' and Holly promptly folded her arms across her chest in a disgruntled manner – a real teenage strop!

Holly, while developmentally delayed, also had the typical moods of adolescence to contend with, it would seem, although the conversation with her was like that of relating to a 3- or 4-year-old. When you are sad, suggested Maddy, you can look at the sad side and remember the rainbow connection, that the rain is part of the rainbow. At this point in the activity, Holly paused and seemed to inhabit a different space and awareness, deeply reflective, for a full four or five seconds, pondering this deep spiritual truth, which she understood perhaps better than anyone else in the room. There would be difficult days, but something shifts and the rainbow appears and the two things are connected. In this moment, Maddy became aware of the spiritual profundity of Holly, something she could sense and see in her posture and being. There was no need to fill that silence, but to marvel simply at this mystical awareness in Holly, the meeting of hearts, and the fact that there was no need to fix, change or fill any gap. Holly, in those precious moments, was leading the way in knowledge and understanding. After this activity and encounter, Holly was suddenly tired and reading the signals, Maddy said, 'Shall we leave you in peace?' They shared a high five, then Holly took Maddy's hand and kissed it before they parted ways.

Maddy Parkes, spiritual care practitioner

Times of distress

Even when a chaplain's presence is not apparently making much impact there is evidence from our experience at BCH that children and young people value the support, acceptance and non-judgemental presence of chaplains during times of distress and illness. The activity, at times, may be of less relevance; however, introducing the activity allows the staff member to be with the young person in a less threatening way, coming alongside to support and encourage. Having something to hold on to and anchor them, a tangible gift representing care and support, can be particularly important for young people navigating ill health. One young person, having survived a serious trauma, received a prayer rope with real gladness and, her parent reported later, insisted on holding this, having it near, or hanging it within her own line of vision. Another child was grateful for a holding cross and commented, 'You always bring me nice things.' Examples of less religious objects given are postcards with pictures and readings, hanging heart mobiles, Easter decorative chicks, decorations for bed spaces, battery operated tea lights. These too can carry spiritual meanings, such as the glowing light in the darkness, the love and importance of relationships or the strength of being connected to others.

Waiting rooms

There can be long periods of waiting when in hospital, in day clinics and on the ward, which can be difficult for parents and children to manage. Offering resources can help to transform a dull period of waiting into a lively interactive encounter, where time flies by and spiritual care takes place. The activities do not have to be complex to be effective.

Threshold moments

On occasion, the activity and involvement with the young person may occur at a point of significant change: the day before or after an operation, a birthday, or the day of discharge from the hospital. One chaplain visited Roberta at the threshold moment of going home: while the family waited for all to be finally in place for leaving that afternoon, the chaplain marked this significant moment of departure by making a bracelet with Roberta. When the bracelet was in place, they held hands, a final prayer was offered and an embrace. After more than a year of pastoral contact, it was fortuitous that this visit happened in the way that it did, contributing to a 'good ending', honouring Roberta's journey through and recognising the significance of relationships and experience, also noting hopes and the anticipation of the future, and all that going home meant.

Threshold moments can also be part of brief and one-off encounters with children in the hospital. For instance, meeting Lara for the first time during a participation day, which happened to be the day of her discharge from hospital, the chaplain nonetheless found that through the activity of making a sensory box, Lara spoke freely about the story of her accident and her worries and hopes about returning to school. Though a fleeting contact, the opportunity to build a reflective space about a significant experience was made through sharing this activity, offering support to a young person going through a significant life experience.

ACTIVITY 6.7: MAKING A JIGSAW

Sam was a bright 7-year-old being treated for cancer and was visiting the day clinic. Bored and restless, he seized the opportunity to make a puzzle. This activity simply requires a blank jigsaw puzzle and some felt pens. Having a degree of challenge was appropriate for this lively minded child – creating a system of ordering the puzzle pieces on the back with numbers and then colouring in a connecting design on the other side. Using stencils created another dimension to the play, and Sam quickly became absorbed in making a boat, with two sides of the sail in distinct colours of red and blue. 'This is me,' he explained, unprompted, pointing to one side of the sail, 'and this is my brother,' pointing to the other. From the outset, Sam was intent on placing a star on the top of his mast, and explained, 'This is my sister.' He looked at the boat and pointed to the four colourful sticky gems he had stuck onto the base of the boat; 'This is my mother, my dad, and my aunties.' 'You have you entire family in the boat,' I suggested. This was a living, active metaphor for Sam which lent itself beautifully to conversation about the importance of family and navigating through choppy waters, but all being in the boat together. In the middle of the encounter, Sam's dad drew a reluctant Sam away to have his check-up, after which Sam returned eagerly to his puzzle making. The spiritual care activity was not distraction therapy; rather, the clinic contact became the distraction from the business of self-reflection, meaning making and creative pursuit.

Rev Kathryn Darby, chaplain

PRACTICE EXAMPLE 6.6: PAULA GOING HOME

Two chaplains sharing in a participation day, approached a 15-year-old girl, Paula, for the first time, introducing themselves and offering some postcards which Paula responded to. Using a Blob Tree illustration, Paula chose the blob figure 'sitting near the top of the trunk, smiling with her arm waving – because she was going home!' We then used a postcard illustrating pathways and asking, 'Which path reminds you most of your life? Why? Draw your own path that you think is like your life…' This prompted Paula to reflect on where she was; she chooses the woodland path 'because there are roots on the ground to trip over' connected with the fact that she was leaving the hospital with crutches, but hinting also at the challenges she faced. When asked what things helped her while in hospital, Paula responded, 'The nurses and people asking you what you want and listening to you.' She is given resources to take away and a visiting card with forget-me-nots around a tree, 'I will not forget you. See I have written your name on my hand…' (Isaiah 49, 15–16). At this threshold moment of leaving the hospital, and during this rather fleeting encounter and episode of pastoral care, the chaplains provided space, reflection time, reassurance, faith connection, and materials for the ongoing journey from hospital back to home, and possibly to church and a confirmation class.

Rev Pamela Turner and Sister Florence Njoku, chaplains

The hospital becomes a context of change, growth, suffering, mystery and significance, and therefore leaving the hospital is complex and may signal grief and loss, as well as relief for children and young people.

PRACTICE EXAMPLE 6.7: SAYING GOODBYE TO JESSICA

Jessica was a very reflective and cognitively able 13-year-old, whose sense of humour and determination had carried her through many difficult hours. We had developed a strong relationship over the many months that she was an in-patient and often, while engaging in different activities, she had shared her concerns and frustrations, family issues and future hopes. The day of discharge finally came and it seemed important to mark the significance of this moment of transition. I offered a selection of beads to make a bracelet, to take away as a gift on her leaving day, and once this activity began, the talking increased! She spoke of her relationships, some of her insecurities and fears, and her plans for the future. A tender moment was shared as I tied the bracelet on to Jessica's wrist with well wishes for her departure. Jessica then offered me her hand to hold, as I spoke a prayer of blessing over her and for her. It was a satisfying ending for me, as I wanted to have the chance to say goodbye properly, and beneficial for Jessica too, who was leaving this significant chapter behind.

Rev Kathryn Darby, chaplain

Simple resources are good

Although we have been talking about some profound encounters we have had, the value of having very simple resources available should not be underestimated. Visiting Jason and his dad on the oncology ward at Easter, and noticing that he was a little restless and that both were feeling cooped up in a small, isolated room, the chaplain said she would go back to the chaplaincy office and collect some books. Among the books and the Easter sticker book for Jason, she picked up a wonderful Noah's ark set. She was as intrigued as Jason to open up and look inside the cardboard boat to reveal the sets of animals in twos, a book and a frieze for his stark hospital bedroom. Everyone's eyes lit up as they explored the toy, but it was especially pleasing to see Jason's spirit become increasingly animated. 'Thank you!' he said repeatedly. Such a boost for all of us! 'You like rainbows, don't you, Jason?' his dad asked, noticing the splendid rainbow that held the toy together like the handles of a bag.

Leaving the ward, the chaplain distributed another sticker book to 4-year-old Vicky; the previous day the chaplain had met her for the first time, sharing sparkling star stickers, and she had later told her mum. 'That lady gave me stickers and I didn't even do anything!' Vicky was pleased to receive this new addition to her collection, and then the chaplain noticed she was carrying one last book that she happened to pick up in her haste to gather a few things together for Jason. It was a small cardboard book with tattered edges and a simple design. Simon, who was next to Vicky, spied the book and said, 'I know that book! That's my favourite book!' and his little body seemed to awaken in anticipation as the chaplain handed it to him. Although he was only 3, he knew all of the words and told her the story confidently as she turned the pages to reveal the fierce lion, the naughty monkey and the scary snake and then the puppy, which was perfect for keeping. His mum told the chaplain that he has that book at home – it really is his favourite – and that they were going home that day but would return one week later for further treatment. Simon was handing the book back to me, having read it through several times, 'I have one at home,' he said solemnly, 'I don't need this one.' 'When you come back next week,' the chaplain suggested, 'I can return with this one and read it with you again.' 'Would you?!' he said in earnest intensity. The promise was made and the book duly stored in safe keeping with Simon's name on it for future meetings, knowing that it is essential to keep promises made to children. There can be a providential feel to the work that we do, where the most tattered book underneath a pile of beautiful resources becomes the treasure in the hands of a small boy, and also the means of meeting together in a real and supportive manner.

There are times when the simplest activities are the most apt for a situation, particularly with the very young. Having a supply of bubbles, for instance, is a useful tool. Visiting on the oncology ward, having bubbles was a direct and effective way to engage with a 14-month-old girl who was somewhat restless, being carried in her mother's arms. It offered distraction but also something more. She became enraptured with the delicate bubbles finding shape and floating before her eyes, squealing with delight, eyes open with wonder. A child can lead us all into a few moments of escape and joy in their ability to enter fully into a moment of awe. Similarly, a 3-year-old child, immobile and held in suspension after a road traffic accident, could laugh and participate in a game, as bubbles were caught and layered, counting them together.

Making flowers or paper chains is a straightforward but pleasing activity that can give children a fairly instant sense of accomplishment and enjoyment. There are times when coming up with a new activity using a few simple materials can be a rewarding antidote to highly sophisticated electronic games, especially when instigated by a child or young person. For instance, Leo (3), seeing colourful string and large stickers, took the lead in designing a mobile with three hearts representing his mum, dad and himself.

Mental health

Self-esteem and trust can be very low, and a fear of failure can be high for children and young people with mental health issues, therefore they might be reluctant to engage in an activity or contact. One senior youth worker suggests, 'CAMHS [Children and Adolescent Mental Health Services] in-patients need time to develop a trusting relationship and means of communication. And yet, creative activities can be a way of protecting the individual against being overwhelmed, for instance, by depression' (Storr in Barritt 2005). There are occasions when spiritual care practitioners are able to build a relationship of trust over time, and using activities can help to generate rapport and engage in a non-threatening way. This was evidenced by the work with Della who, after a stay in hospital over a period of several months in which regular contact was given, gave us a card when she left the hospital which said, simply, 'Thank you for being there when I wanted to talk.' Such developed relationships are not always possible, nonetheless, there is scope, even in a brief encounter, to offer trust and care, and such genuine gifts are often welcomed at some level by any person who is going through a difficult time.

Joanne Stevens, a CAMHS nurse, adapted activities that chaplaincy had developed for spiritual care for use with her patients (see Appendix 2). Aware that children and young people with mental health issues were moving through the ward fairly rapidly once assessment and treatment plans were made, she wanted to maximise the help that she could offer. Some weeks later, she reported how using these tools helped her make connections and build trust with young people, leading to four separate disclosures about very serious issues. This stresses the need for understanding safeguarding and referral policies and procedures.

PRACTICE EXAMPLE 6.8: NATHANIEL'S EASTER STORY BRACELET

Nathaniel (10) eagerly welcomed the opportunity to make an Easter story bracelet with me, although this proved to be one of only two instances of contact, as he was transferred. However, in the relatively brief encounter, Nathaniel and I built a rapport, and he enjoyed the activity, which focused his mind on the Easter story and the presence of Christ at the tomb, appearing to Mary. While going through his own 'darkness of the soul' and eating disorder connected with bullying, there was opportunity to connect with his faith narrative and the strength of belonging to a faith community, and with the message that God was with him, as well as offering a supportive presence for the parents. Nathaniel was honest and open about his sadness and his troubles, as well as his sources of hope. He made something that he was proud to wear and to show his parents at a time in his life when his self-esteem was low.

Rev Kathryn Darby, chaplain

Carers: Demands on carers of children with mental health issues

Providing spiritual care for children and young people with mental health difficulties can place different kinds of strains on the carer. The boundaries of what is 'normal' are fluid, and encountering another human being whose sense of inner isolation, alienation and distress is acute makes particular demands upon those offering support, as their own sense of meaning and identity is challenged. This can apply both to family members and staff. Feeling disconcerted may be an inevitable part of truly entering the world of another person who feels confusion, fear and uncertainty and even deep existential alienation (Carson 2008, p.53). Carers need to remain grounded, nurturing their own spiritual connectedness and resilience, as the inner world experience of the person may include crisis and terror (Carson 2008). Particularly in relation to psychotic experience, the usual pastoral components of empathy and congruence may not be as relevant as 'loyalty, tolerance and practical caring' (Carson 2008, p.56). 'Authenticity' in listening, telling and reinterpreting stories, which form the fabric of human identity, is also essential (Robinson, Kendrick and Brown 2003), and relates closely to the chaplain's ongoing self-reflection.

Working with groups can offer
a wider or shared meaning

While significant amounts of spiritual care are done one-to-one, there are times when a group activity can be helpful.

ACTIVITY 6.8: 3D BLOB TREE

Together with the play and youth work department, chaplaincy designed a project running for three weeks in the summer holidays, funded by BCH Charities, inviting children and young people to shape a blob figure out of clay, approximately 10 cm high, to represent themselves at that particular time. During a blob-making session with Josefina (15), who was recovering from severe burns, Melissa (15), being treated for cystic fibrosis, and Arron (15), who was being assessed with mental health difficulties, the young people were able to relax into a conversation about their conditions, the challenges and their attitudes to life, and their sense of attachment to the hospital. Melissa designed a blob in a wheelchair, reflecting her own state of mobility at that stage. Arron, whose self-esteem and trust in adults was low, created a surfing figure. Other blobs reflected physical features and moods – thoughtful, happy, sad, adventurous, perplexed – which were brought together and placed on a blob tree and displayed in the hospital corridor. Leaves were designed for the tree, using copper, and words and messages relating to being in hospital for others were inscribed on the leaves (see Appendix 2 for instructions). Children and young people who were not able to attend the session could create one at their bed.

Charlotte Frith, youth worker

Opportunities also occur to work with small groups of children in play rooms, adolescent rooms, or, when they were within reach of one another, on a ward. Group dynamics allow for a less intense way of working, and at times the chaplain can facilitate and encourage interaction and conversation between young people, building community and allowing more reticent members of the group to feel included and affirmed. However, it can be helpful for some children and young people to take part in a wider project even if they can't join the group. Thus, in his ongoing work with Mandy (15), who was receiving spinal surgery and had a history of self-harm and mental health issues, the youth worker left clay for her to make a blob figure. Returning for another visit, it was evident that the 'blob' task had led to reflection for Mandy and she spoke candidly about her experience using the language of hope. She had made two blob characters, one looking sad, and the other with a hoody on it using a mobile phone. Mandy explained how the second blob was 'hiding in her hood but using her phone to get help and support', revealing her coping strategies, which led to further discussion about developing resilience. It was appropriate to offer a chapel visit, which Mandy valued.

PRACTICE EXAMPLE 6.9: FACILITATING PEER SUPPORT

Working in groups can facilitate peer support, as one youth worker describes of his work with Bonny and Ethan. Making blob figures draws them into conversation. 'I turned to Bonny and asked her what blob she was making to represent how she felt. She had picked up a black piece of modelling clay and was making what she described as a ghost. She said she was afraid, as she was due to have an operation which she had never had before. At this point I leaned towards Ethan and asked if he would have any advice to give to Bonny. Ethan told Bonny that he had had a lot of operations before and that there wasn't anything to be afraid of. He asked her if she was having laughing gas and told her that would make things better.' Ethan went on to offer other reassurances built on his own experiences. 'Bonny really took this on board, she smiled and changed her ghost when showing other young people.' The youth worker was surprised. 'Due to Ethan having ASD he is normally quite hyperactive and rarely holds conversations with other young people. So for him to actually engage with a young person and reassure them at the same time definitely was not what I expected.'

Dave Baker, youth worker

Many of the activities described in this book could be used with groups, but being mindful of the capacity of children and young people to engage is important. It may be that several spiritual care practitioners are needed to provide support for those who cannot do the activity on their own. What can also be useful are normalising activities where children and young people may get to talk about life outside of hospital and perhaps engage in a discussion, which may be similar to something they might do at school or a club.

ACTIVITY 6.9: MY FAVOURITE DAY

Sometimes activities can facilitate meaning making in groups. This activity is aimed at helping children and young people visualise an ideal day. Through doing this they can perhaps recognise what is truly important to them and/or what gives them joy. I have done this with children and young people from 7 to 18 using both written and/or oral response. I have found it works better to encourage written answers followed by oral sharing. Some of them may need assistance in reading and writing. Or, in cases where written language skills are severely lacking, encouragement to provide oral only responses may be in order.

Begin by inviting an honest discussion of what it is like to be confined to the hospital and unable to go home. Sometimes I start by saying that I have tried to imagine what it must be like for them and, although I can try to put myself in their place (in my mind), I still don't really know what it must feel like. And then I ask them, 'What is it like for you? What do you miss?' After we talk about that for a short time, I tell them, 'Today we are going to use our imagination to describe our "perfect" day. I have some questions to help us imagine. There are no right or wrong answers. YOUR answer is the best answer (for you)!'

Hand out the questions and give everyone time to answer them:

1. Where are you?

2. Who is with you?

3. What are you doing?

4. What kind of day is it?

5. What are you wearing?

6. Is there food? What kind?

7. What is the most important part of the day for you?

8. Who, besides you, will remember this day?

9. How does this day change you?

10. Could this day happen in real life?

11. What would it take for this day to happen?

When everyone has finished, call them back to the circle. At this point you have two options for sharing the information:

1. You can have each person, one by one, read all their answers in order. The advantage of this method is you get the whole picture (image) of what that person's favourite day would be like. In groups where the majority of participants have a moderately good attention span, this is the best way to share. However, if participants do not have good attention skills, find it hard to listen to others, or are restless, option b) works better.

2. Going around the circle, have each participant provide their answer to each question. For example, the first person would say where they are on their favourite day. Then the next person, going around the circle, would say who is with them on this favourite day. And so on. An advantage of this method is that it is easier to see the similarities and contrasts in the different participant's day – who is inside or outside, who is at home or on a beach or at an amusement park, how many people have their family with them, etc. The harder part, of course, is for the facilitator to put together the full image of any one individual participant's day. This can be easily compensated for by asking the participant to let you look for a minute at their page to see it all together.

Rev Kristin Moore, chaplain

Spiritual care for professionals

Reciprocity can be an important element of spiritual care, recognising that the spiritual care practitioner is also on a journey of spiritual growth and discovery. While the encounter should remain child centred, the spiritual care practitioner may be affected and sometimes surprised by the impact of the encounter on them and the resonances with their own spiritual life. One chaplain observes that there was a shared 'sense of vitality and delight' and the 'whole meeting had a sense of encounter in Christ' when reflecting on a spiritual care encounter. Various spiritual care practitioners comment on the encouragement they received through the creative process of engaging with activities and watching children and young people respond and perhaps developing rapport with others through a shared activity. Reflecting on the balance between 'doing to' and 'doing with' is important, including knowing when 'doing with' is a more appropriate choice in an awareness of the child's level of vulnerability which may be involved in this. Spiritual care practitioners are often awestruck by what children say and share, facing the challenge of illness with a generosity of spirit and a positive attitude, perseverance, humour and a welcoming attitude. For instance, drawing alongside Ria, whose cerebral palsy affects her fine motor skills, the chaplain was repeatedly encouraged to accept her own limitations. While there were spills and smudges, Ria would remark happily: 'It doesn't really matter!' In entering the world of play the spiritual care practitioner may be surprised at their own reactions and responses and needs to have appropriate places to reflect and review. This is something which BCH chaplaincy do as a team and also offer to other teams or departments within the hospital.

Summary

Helping children and young people to make sense of the often difficult and demanding time in hospital can be a vital part of effective spiritual care.

- Metaphors may help children and young people explore spiritual life and engage with mystery and human experience.

- Activities help young people to process their experience or prepare for going home.

- Offering spiritual care activities in groups can facilitate meaning making amongst peers.

- Being inventive with simple materials to suit individuals can be an effective approach.

- The products of spiritual care need to be treated with respect and reverence and children and young people empowered to make choices as to what happens to them.

- For some, an act of spiritual care will have more meaning, depth and richness if it is an act of religious care.

Chapter 7

Spiritual Care with Families

PRACTICE EXAMPLE 7.1: WORKING WITH MIA

Mia (2) had been through tremendous challenges, moving with her family recently from South Africa and diagnosed with a relapse of cancer. Her two older brothers were attending the hospital school, and were navigating life in hospital in a new culture and environment. When Mia first arrived on the ward, her parents were in a state of shock and confusion. She held on tightly to her mum and did not want much contact with me, showing real reluctance to engage. The parents were Christians and eager for a prayer to be said. Holding hands and gathering around Mia, I noticed that during the time of prayer, Mia became more upset, perhaps picking up on the distress of her parents, and possibly feeling crowded by this gathering of adults around her, including me, whose face was new to her. I went away feeling dispirited about the prayer and the initial 'failed' contact with a vulnerable child.

Gradually, over time, I gained Mia's trust, offering her little opportunities to play and showing an interest in her. On one occasion I created a diverting scene with a hand puppet while the doctor tried to address the concerns of Mia's mother and on another by offering Mia some stickers and some pretty paper flowers at a moment when she was brought very low in condition and spirits. At another time, I intrigued Mia with a pesky toy animal. In these small ways, I sought to communicate

---

care, fun and friendliness. The activities and materials for engaging with Mia became immensely important in bridging a large gulf created by change, illness and the discomforts of treatment.

I happened upon Mia and her dad one day in the play room. Mia was upset, and Dad was attempting to comfort her. She was asking for her mummy who had gone out to run an errand. I reached into my bag for a sticker book and Mia soon became distracted by this colourful book of stickers. The tears were wiped away as she began to put the stickers on the page and talk about where she wanted to place the pictures. She became cheerful again and quietly absorbed in her activity. Together, we made an Easter bracelet. 'I can show Mummy!' she said in her chirping voice, and her daddy and I both encouraged her. Doing this simple stilling exercise enabled Mia to calm down, and to be assured that her mummy would return to her. I remembered what Mia's mother had told me on another occasion, that Mia loved her brothers and enjoyed seeing them. 'Will you also show your brothers what you have been making?' I asked. 'Yes,' she agreed, 'I will show them.' Prior to this particular meeting with Mia, trust had already been built over a period of weeks, enabling me to settle in quickly with the activity. Our relationship had moved a long way from that initial visit when Mia was wary of every stranger and hiding her face in her mother's arm. When it was time to go, Mia's dad said, 'Thank you. You came at exactly the right time.' The timing and possibilities for that contact were only possible because of my previous painstaking efforts to build rapport with a small and bewildered person trying to make sense of her changing world.

At times the chemotherapy treatment had left Mia very ill and unsettled, and in turn the family were distressed, although they took strength in their faith. Mum appreciated the prayers and blessing and receiving chaplaincy cards, with encouraging reflections and pictures and reminders of her faith, and the children enjoyed being part of the hospital school community, taking part in the Christmas service in the chapel and getting to know adults and children who cared for them. But they had all experienced a sense of dislocation and upheaval, and the treatment journey was not over yet. Eventually, they became settled in a local community and appreciated the ongoing links with chaplaincy, including advice and support in finding a church home and community links.

Rev Kathryn Darby, chaplain

Assessment and intervention

Families assemble in various shapes and sizes and may include a single parent or more than one set of parents, heterosexual or same-sex partners, extended family of grandparents, aunts and uncles and cousins, and importantly, siblings, all of whom may frequently appear at the bedside or may be relating from a distance. But the entire family is significant to the child and it is important to help the child to make connections within the context of family in order to accentuate the support that is there.

ACTIVITY 7.1: HOPE BLANKET

The Hope Blanket (see Appendix 2) project involved gathering individual squares of cotton, painted and designed by children, young people and their families, to make a quilt that went on display outside of the chapel, exploring the theme, 'Hopes and Dreams'. Families could enjoy their own artwork, bound with colourful ribbon to the squares of other families, together forming a beautiful tapestry.

The presence and support of family for a child or young person who is sick is essential and pivotal to the care that a spiritual care practitioner brings. Most often spiritual care practitioners relate to the whole family. Treatment in hospital can lead to huge family disruption, separation, and the challenge for parents who have to balance life in two places – home and hospital – and may feel torn when they are in one place or the other. Spiritual care can be about helping parents to let go of idealised notions and high expectations about themselves as parents: 'good enough' can be liberating. Activities with children can ease the way to a significant contact with their parent or carer. While providing a point of connection with children and young people, engaging in activities may also lead parents to decide that the chaplain or spiritual care practitioner is a 'safe person', as their interactions with their child are observed.

PRACTICE EXAMPLE 7.2: SIONED AND HER DAD

I met Sioned (5) and her dad for the first time during a routine visit on the ward, when an initial smile and introduction were exchanged. I offered Sioned a heart sticker, which matched the heart design on her top, and gave her some paper to make a picture. When Sioned's dad needed to step off the ward for a short time, I stayed with Sioned, completing the picture, and then offered another activity. In the process, I began to access Sioned's ability, which had evidently been affected by her brain tumour. Dad confirmed upon his return that Sioned had lost much of her sight through cancer. As the activities were completed, Dad asked for a private conversation, drawing the curtain around the bed and initiating a discussion about his loss of faith, the anguish of crying out to God, 'Why my child?' and the nature of heaven. He had a pressing question. 'Will my child be blind in heaven?' While he was angry with God about the circumstances of Sioned's life, he welcomed this opportunity for an honest conversation about coping with cancer and his wrestling with faith. All of this sprang from an initial greeting and a time of engaging with spiritual care activities. A promise was made to make further contact and I explained about the location of the chapel in the hospital as a significant place of refuge.

Rev Kathryn Darby, chaplain

We have developed spiritual care resources which offer a focus for the whole family to relate to one another, strengthening communication and care for the child who is ill and also facilitating families in being more present to, and aware of, each other. Sometimes parents who have become familiar with and trusting of the chaplain or spiritual care practitioner will seize the opportunity when they approach to take a break away from the bedside. It can be extremely confining for the parent who is tied to the bed space, and they will value a chance to make a phone call, take a shower, have a short walk or simply a stretch and a rest away from their intense role of caring one-on-one for their child. When they are ill, children and young people will likely need more emotional support and appear almost to regress in their development, wanting their mum or dad to be in close proximity. Parents will want to fulfil this desire, but this can also be highly demanding and exhausting.

ACTIVITY 7.2: SIMPLE QUESTIONNAIRES

Sometimes with families introducing something as a simple questionnaire can facilitate conversation between them. This can be adapted to explore many different issues. One example had three questions: What do you like about being in hospital? What do you miss by being away from home? Is there anything we could do about it? This set of questions opened up a lively dialogue between a father and son, Tom (6), being treated on the cardiac ward. A strong interaction developed between the child and his father, as Tom expressed his longing for home, his dog and a restored sense of normality. While these issues might be commonly understood by adults as a necessary hardship for the sake of getting better, giving a young child opportunity to articulate their needs and their sense of loss along the way can be immensely important. After the discussion, Tom's dad expressed his gladness that they had 'thought these issues out well'.

Rev Nick Ball, chaplain

The hospital family

Attachments are also formed in the hospital – with staff, other families, wards and routines – and a temporary new home and an extended sense of family may be established. For some families, whose child has been in hospital since infancy and may have a long stay, the hospital becomes like a second home. Nurses and support staff, and teachers and allied professionals particularly build up important and strong relationships with children and young people and are very important members of their circle of care. Christmas 2014 offered a good example of the way some children feel a continuing attachment to their hospital family. Several years on from her successful kidney transplant, Priyanka and her mum arrived at the annual renal ward nativity service with a very large box of samosas to share and a card and present for Paul. The family are Muslims, and Priyanka and Paul talked about the contract they had when she was in hospital: he would pray for her if she would pray for him, reflecting reciprocity, spiritual care across faith boundaries and a sense of belonging to the renal ward family, which celebrates Christmas each year with a nativity. This time it was a *Frozen* theme where they were looking for a king not a queen!

PRACTICE EXAMPLE 7.3: MIRIUM'S BEADS

The chaplain approached Mirium (14) who was being treated for cystic fibrosis and welcomed the offer to make a 'Who loves and cares for me' bracelet, an adaptation of the original idea. The chaplain hoped that the activity might enable the young person to reflect on how many different people care for her at a time when she was removed from her usual support network. The bracelet would be a tangible way of being aware of these people and things in her life. Mirium took the beads and sorted them into piles of similar-sized beads, as the chaplain explained that the different beads could represent anything or anyone that made her feel loved and cared for, suggesting that Mirium might consider family members, friends, school, community and extra-curricular groups. Mirium chose beads for specific people in her life and told the chaplain about each one, testing the chaplain's memory each time a new bead was added. She was eager to share her reasons for representing people with the beads and also chose several beads associated with her cystic fibrosis. As each bead was added, Mirium repeated who and what each bead represented, and once completed showed the bracelet to other patients and staff, explaining the meaning and delighting in the process.

Zamir Hussain, chaplain

Families will often talk about their hospital family and the way in which staff become a significant part of their family experience, particularly those who spend long periods in hospital and whose wider family may live a considerable distance away or are simply not involved. We try in our spiritual care activities to express some of this connectedness to the hospital family, as well as their own family.

ACTIVITY 7.3: FAMILY CARING TREE

We have been working with Victoria Beech of God Venture (www. godventure.co.uk) to develop some resources for work with families. One of these is the family caring tree, which is one way to bring the focus of the family to the fore and identify the important people who are in a child's life but may not be in close proximity. Chaplain Rachel Hill-Brown describes how she showed Wilf, who had been in the hospital for virtually all of his two-and-a-half years of life, the family tree card and talked about who was in Wilf's family. He chose the stickers he wanted for each family member and placed them on the card himself, telling Rachel who each person was and asking her to draw hair on each of them. The names were written on the card and then the words spoken, 'Thank you God for...' Saying 'thank you' for Wilf made him grin broadly.

Although Wilf could not speak due to a tracheotomy he could communicate very clearly with signs and pointed to pictures in his language book. This activity was a wonderful opportunity for Wilf to express himself – his likes/dislikes – and opened up discussion. Mum then asked him who else cares. He was reluctant initially so Mum suggested nurses. He shook his head, so Mum listed some names and he chose one of his favourite nurses and then chose a sticker to put on the card. Mum then asked about others who care and listed a few. Wilf chose the physiotherapist and stuck a sticker on for her. Mum then suggested a doctor. Wilf was adamant that he did not want a doctor on his caring card. Mum talked to him about the different doctors whom he sees and eventually he was happy to include one that he liked. The caring card showed how Wilf found some aspects of life in hospital a challenge, revealing perhaps resentment and anger at some of what he has had to endure in hospital. It was noticeable also when Wilf did not want certain figures to feature on his caring card. This was slightly uncomfortable for his mum and the chaplain because of the desire to make things as good as possible for Wilf, and having to face the reality that he was affected by some of the less pleasant things he has had to endure.

Wilf loved doing these cards and some weeks later he still had them attached to the end of his bed, showing them to the chaplain on several occasions. The cards also became a talking point with his mum, and a further way of sharing this important awareness of family with one another. Together with Wilf, his mum made a small picture album with photographs of family, significant carers, friends and extended community, which he would often reach for and consider with her. This aspect of spiritual care – understanding that we belong to and are valued within a family group was further enabled by the chaplain and the family resources.

These activities helped the adults to affirm Wilf and his place within his family and helped Wilf to communicate about how important his family was to him, his love for them and his sense of belonging and connectedness.

Rev Rachel Hill-Brown, chaplain

Siblings

Some activities, such as card making, can facilitate young people in relating to their siblings even when they are not present. One small girl was happy for the opportunity to design her own card which, she decided was 'for her brother because she missed him'. Particularly for those children who have to spend long periods in isolation due to their low immunity or to the concern about passing on infections – such as this 3-year-old who was receiving treatment for cancer – there can be a real pain and loss in being taken out of their usual home environment, missing the comforts of home and the companionship of siblings. Noticeably, very small children often light up with joy when their older sister or brother comes to visit. Siblings are going through their own spiritual journey. They may be feeling bored, neglected, anxious, angry, frustrated, lonely, fearful. The post-operation time can be a worrying one for a sibling, as it may seem that what was meant to make a sister or brother better has in fact made him or her feel worse. The challenges can be intensified for a child when the birth of their brother or sister seems to result in separating them more from their parent who needs to be with the new sibling in hospital. Offering reassurance, affirmation and hope can be important things to share with siblings at this difficult time.

PRACTICE EXAMPLE 7.4: IN THE BEREAVEMENT SUITE

Parents, grandparents and sibling, Daniel, of a baby who just died were all in the Rainbow room to spend time with the child. I saw that it was important to distract Daniel with a play activity, so that the rest of the family had the opportunity to spend time with their baby in a focused way knowing that Daniel was being well cared for. I found some play dough in the cupboard and this developed into a spiritual care encounter. Daniel made shapes and then flattened the circle of dough into a face with a sad expression. I asked, 'What would make the sad expression a happy face?' 'I could go swimming with Mummy,' Daniel suggested, doing the actions of swimming with his play dough sad face, getting really involved in the imaginative play. Together we changed the expression on the face, from sad to happy. By engaging with Daniel I helped the rest of the family meet their own spiritual care needs. My reflection is that children don't always have the words; we need to find tools to get into their world.

Sally Roberts, family support play worker

At the same time, spending time at hospital with their family can lead to positive experiences for the siblings as they also become valued members of a diverse community. Spiritual care practitioners can offer a great deal in this regard. Involving siblings in spiritual care activities can be a way of including them, making them feel special, giving them loving attention, offering a positive hospital experience, giving them expression for a range of feelings and helping them to process their experience, build community and family solidarity. Siblings, including the child who is sick, may welcome the opportunity to make something for the sister or brother that they love, are concerned about or are forced to spend long periods separated from. For instance, 3-year-old Emily (being treated for cancer) chooses to make a bookmark for her older brother, while her sisters, Lisa and Molly (7 and 4 years old), happily make a card and a picture for their baby brother who is on the intensive care ward.

PRACTICE EXAMPLE 7.5: SARA'S DREAM SPACE

Elsie offered the Dream Space activity to 14-year-old Sara. After spending some quiet moments thinking, Sara said, 'I know what I want to draw, but I don't know how' and then burst into tears. The nurses instantly descended, asking 'Is everything all right?' and Elsie offered reassurances before helping Sara to express the difficult feelings she was living with. Sara explained that her brother would soon be leaving for university and she was worried about him. With Elsie's help, she made a picture of this important time of change in her life: a house is framed at the bottom of the picture and a university is framed at the top corner. Elsie suggested drawing a path between these two places, which could include pictures and symbols of Sara's feelings and concerns, those things that are difficult to carry, using stickers. Sara chose two people to walk on the path, and also some sad faces, one with a great outpouring of tears and emotion. Some sticker people, representing family, were stuck above the home. Amidst the signs of sadness and grief Sara chose other stickers: a heart, a green shrub, a butterfly and a star in the sky. It is important that children are given scope to explore both the light and dark within the hospital experience, but this needs to be done with sensitivity in a way that offers some closure and containment.

With sensitivity and pastoral awareness, Elsie enabled Sara to express and process her difficult emotions as well as providing symbols of hope: the road and the sense of connection this provided, the presence of brother, sister and family in relationship, the symbols of life in the sky. Elsie listened to the important feelings, created a safe space for Sara to explore and contain these feelings, and led her into a place of greater resolution.

Rev Elsie Blair-Chappell, chaplain

It can be difficult for siblings who, visiting a sick brother or sister, must endure the confines of a small bed space, with little to do, and where the attention is necessarily on the sick child. Involving siblings in spiritual care activities can be a way of building a positive experience in an often stressful and distressing circumstance, which in turn will support the child who is sick, especially if activities can be shared.

ACTIVITY 7.4: PAPER FLOWERS

Sometimes simplifying the focus, and using easily accessible materials such as a little paper and a bit of sticky tape can open up the broader spaces between people and within the soul. As part of an Easter theme, we made flowers with children out of paper cupcake holders, brightly coloured pipe cleaners and bead centres. Leaves were cut out of green paper, and each element of the flower woven onto the pipe cleaner in turn. Using a drop of essential oil of lavender in the centre of the flower added an extra sensory dimension. Children of all ages and their parents and carers enjoyed making these flowers which could then wrap around bed frames to brighten up bed spaces, bringing people together to make something simple and beautiful, opening up conversation and contacts, and reminding us all of the delights and colours of nature.

Eleana woke up on the intensive care ward after a surgery on her airways and was in a state of grogginess and discomfort. The arrival of her three siblings brought energy and joy into the room for Eleana who smiled and evidently wanted them near to her. I introduced a simple craft – making tissue flowers – which the children could all enjoy and share in, entertaining Eleana and creating a colourful focus for the room. The clinical space soon resembled a play room with bright materials brought out onto the bed and children busy making things. Eleana seemed to thrive on this interaction, taking part in small ways and enjoying the activity of her family around her. Her older sister made a flower for Eleana, carefully consulting her about colour and choice of materials, modelling good spiritual care for the adults!

Rev Kathryn Darby, chaplain

Children and young people with additional needs

Accepting young people as they are, particularly if illness or surgery has resulted in a learning disability, physical disability or mobility impairment, is immensely important. When relating to children, it is important to approach them as unique individuals with their own blend of talents and characteristics, keeping pre-judgements in check; a child or young person with physical or mental disabilities is no exception to this. In any encounter, we need to start with them as individuals, rather than the disability or ability.

PRACTICE EXAMPLE 7.6: BECKY'S SENSORY BOX

Becky (13) had suffered a setback after an operation to remove a benign brain tumour. Although making a good recovery, Becky's speech and motor control had been slow to return. Taking materials for sensory boxes onto the neurological ward one day, we gave Becky a box to decorate which she took a great deal of care and time over. She needed some support from me and from her mum but Becky enjoying herself immensely and took evident pride in her work as she posed for a photo. Clearly, her self-esteem had been boosted and her motor skills were also being exercised in the process. It might have first appeared that Becky did not have the co-ordination or readiness to make a sensory box, as her communication was still limited, but this became a wonderful opportunity to break through any such appearances or false conclusions.

Rev Kathryn Darby, chaplain

Developmental issues which are the result of physical or mental disabilities will be running alongside typical development for some children and young people. Delayed development is simply typical development but delayed. A child with severe physical disabilities may have age-appropriate cognitive abilities. Likewise, a child or young person with learning disabilities may well have age-appropriate physical maturity.

Where there is a recognised condition such as autism or ADHD (attention deficit and hyperactivity disorder), some social and communication development may be affected. For instance, a child or young person with autism may offer little verbal communication but have a high cognitive ability. Alternatively, they may exhibit good communication skills but lack social awareness or have very specific routine needs. It is important to relate to each young person individually and seek guidance from them or their main carer as appropriate. The invisibility of some disabilities raises other challenges. For instance, brain tumours can remain undetected in a child for months and even years, causing developmental delay, and when they are removed, adjustment and adaptation is needed by the child and family.

It is also important to note that the new diagnosis of a disability (whether congenital or due to accident or illness) may well cause a process of grief for the child and their carer, even while the child can return to physical health. For instance, a diagnosis of autism is often not made until years after birth. Carers may grieve for the child they thought they had, while they may also appreciate a diagnosis to aid their understanding and care of their child. Children with a sudden physical disability may grieve about their dream of becoming a sports person and may fear the loss of their social network when they return home.

PRACTICE EXAMPLE 7.7: MADDY'S TRIP TO HOSPITAL

Chaplain, Rachel Hill-Brown, whose daughter, Maddy, has Down syndrome, talks about the frustration she feels when people do not wait to see what Maddy can do before jumping to conclusions about her. For instance, Maddy can do many things that other children – with or without disabilities – her age (6) are unable to do. There is a list of top ten likely distinctive features for a child with Down syndrome but any child could have one or more of these. Says Rachel, 'I want the staff to expect the best of my child and not making assumptions; start with high expectations and then adjust them.' Instead of relying on looks or labels it is most helpful to ask: does your child have any medical needs or special needs?

Rachel reflected on her recent experience of bringing Maddy to hospital: 'Staff were good at talking to Maddy first and giving her the opportunity to answer for herself, rather than going directly to me for information. The doctor had explained the procedure to Maddy that was going to take place that morning, and then asked, 'Maddy, do you have any questions?' Maddy replied, 'Yes, what wobbles in the sky?' The doctor looked at her expectantly; answer: 'a Jellycopter!' While not relating directly to the matter of the imminent procedure, Maddy was given opportunity and space, respect and consideration, and chose at that moment to lighten the atmosphere with some humour.

Rev Rachel Hill-Brown, chaplain

As with all children, giving some sense of choice, empowerment and control can be very positive – and we need to find creative ways to do this when the ability of the child is severely limited. With a very physically limited child, for instance, asking them to choose by looking at a specific picture can be effective. Sometimes we have to take risks and try things, particularly when a child's verbal communication is limited, while remaining vigilant and observant about response and ongoing assent.

Parents, understandably, can be highly protective and even defensive, so that high skills in discernment are called for in determining the best approach, using a combination of being child led and gauging the parent's response, which may offer help and direction. Wilf's story above about the family caring tree is a positive example of such an engagement.

PRACTICE EXAMPLE 7.8: SIAN'S PAINTING

Going to see Sian (14) with material for the Dream Space activity, I was not certain about her ability to engage with the activity. When possible, it is advisable to gain understanding from the nursing team; however, this is not always convenient or possible before the spiritual care contact is made. It was evident on first meeting that Sian's mental ability was below a typical range, her speech was delayed, and she was standing with the aid of a body brace. The best way to find out more specifically what she could do was to ask. Her dad who was watching the proceedings from the other side of the bed space suggested, for instance, that I might handle the scissors. Working with children and young people of all abilities requires an ongoing assessment, including when to guide and support in order to encourage and enable, and when to withdraw in order to create sufficient challenge and promote independence.

Sian wanted to paint and needed help positioning and holding her canvas, and also applying the paint to her brush. She asked, 'What do I do?' but it was important to let her know that whatever she wanted to do and was able to do was welcome. Once we got started applying things to the canvas, her dad commented, 'It's amazing, Sian, how you get others to do all the work,' indicating that I may have been underestimating Sian's ability. In the end, she created a wonderful abstract picture using purple and yellow splashes of colour. 'Shall I write your name on?' her dad enquired and we all admired the final result. She was immensely pleased with her picture and said, 'I can put it on my wall at home!' Although I had explained that the canvases were being collected for a joint display, and I tentatively asked if she would like hers to be included, I also could see that the more likely conclusion was that it would travel home with her within the week.

Rev Kathryn Darby, chaplain

The complex nature of loss for families

When responding to families whose child has a disability or is developing disabilities as a disease progresses, it is important to consider the particular needs that may be emerging. Reflecting on her experience as the parent of a child who battled with cancer from the age of 11 and whose condition led to multiple aspects of disability, Liz Bryson suggests that such families are living with complex aspects of loss. An unfolding picture brings the realisation that their child will not have experiences similar to those of most other children and families. In a sense, there is an ongoing experience of 'a living bereavement' and the process of identity loss for both parent or carer and child. Dealing with disability compounded by illness, particularly when that illness is chronic or life limiting, can be a 'painfully long road'. The long haul is often unappreciated or misunderstood by others, leading frequently to isolation and alienation. Parents may lack their own personal space or fail to have their own needs met while always caring for a dependent child, yet within the vulnerability of sickness, a child craves the security of being close to their parent or carer. While struggling to support their child, other demands can seem relentless: fighting for provision within healthcare, education, finance, and social services as well as social spheres including church or faith community. As a consequence, parents can become physically, emotionally and spiritually drained and may well benefit from joining in with whole family spiritual care activities. Given these realities, attention to the spiritual care needs of a young person with disabilities can make an tremendous difference in the life of that family who may be in desperate need of hope and understanding, help in making choices, a safe place to unload, practical support in building resilience and renewal, someone to share their loss with, compassion, care and emotional support.

PRACTICE EXAMPLE 7.9:
MULTIDISCIPLINARY WORKING

Margaret and Jodie visited Sameena (11) who Jodie knew well from previous visits. Margaret had not met the family before, but learnt that Sameena's dad, Mohammed, was the main carer for his two children who both had significant disabilities. While Jodie engaged with Sameena, Margaret struck up a conversation with Mohammed who was sitting quietly in the corner of the isolated room. Noticing her clerical collar, Mohammed asked, 'Are you a priest?' A lively and philosophical conversation developed between them, as he recalled a trip home to India and a vivid memory of looking at the starlit heavens, and shared the meaning of his faith, while enquiring also about Margaret's faith and beliefs. While having to give up his work, Mohammed observed that it was a far greater work to be able to care for his two daughters. As the conversation ended, a note of mutual respect and understanding had been struck between the father and the chaplain. After leaving the room, Jodie commented, 'I now understand what you chaplains do…you certainly covered some important ground!' Meanwhile, Jodie had been able to work in a dedicated way with Sameena.

Rev Margaret Robinson, chaplain and Jodie Cotterrell, play facilitator

---

Helping with bereavement and loss

Books and images can help siblings begin to understand bereavement and loss. One day the intensive care support worker asked for a book to help explain the loss of his brother to a young sibling, Abdul. He had been confused and angry about the death of his newborn brother, affected also by the distress of his parents. By reading a book, *We Will Meet Again in Jannah* (Hussain 2013), which related to the child in his faith tradition and finding a framework for understanding his loss, the child was greatly reconciled and became more peaceful within himself. Feelings of hostility and agitation were eased and he expressed feelings of gratitude, friendship and even joy.

PRACTICE EXAMPLE 7.10: WATCHING SAM AND HIS SPECIAL BOOK WITH HARRY

A Christian family expressed deep concern of how to explain that Harry's baby sister was going to die very shortly. Harry was about 5 and his parents were very concerned with how to explain what was happening with his sister. We could tell this was distracting them from dealing with their own grief. We offered some of the books our Paediatric Chaplaincy Network (www.paediatric-chaplaincy-network.org) had written. The dad said he would like Harry to have *Sam and his Special Book* from the Held in Hope series and asked us to tell it to him. I explained we also had online videos of the book and we could play this to him. Dad gladly accepted.

We met Harry and explained we had some short films that were about children like his sister and would he like to watch one. His sister was in one of our cubicles so we were able to watch the video while the rest of his family were spending time with his sister. The stories are beautifully illustrated and on the video they are sensitively read by the adventurer Bear Grylls. We watched *Sam and his Special Book*, where a child knows he has a life-limited illness and wonders what his room in heaven will be like. As Harry and I watched the video together, I could see out of the corner of my eye the family peering around to see what we were watching, and the longer we watched the more engrossed they became too.

When we finished watching the video, I asked Harry if he now knew this was how poorly his sister was, and after a short pause, he said yes. I asked him what his sister's room might be like in heaven and he told me that it was like the one his mum and dad had made at home, with lots of nice pictures of animals. I explained that we had another film but his time the story would stop and ask him questions. He said he would like to see it, so we watched the same video, except this time, the story would occasionally stop and another voice would come in and ask Harry questions, like, 'Do you know someone like this?' 'How do you feel about Sam?' As Harry answered all the questions, I continued to observe his family become quieter and more attentive to what was happening on the screen and to Harry's responses. When we finished watching the second video, I asked Harry if he would like to help me do something nice for his sister. He gladly and willing said yes. So he stood holding my plate of gold hearts for his family to take one and place them on his sister, and then placed one on her himself.

Rev Paul Nash, chaplain

At BCH we are developing a range of faith-based resources for children and young people and their parents (email rbr@bch.nhs.uk for details).

PRACTICE EXAMPLE 7.11: SPIRITUAL
CARE FOR BEREAVED FAMILIES

Although this book is not directly about bereavement, some of the children and young people we look after do not get better, and our support to the family continues after their child has died. Many hospitals, hospices and support organisations have wanted to support families who may not have any particular religious beliefs. This was also the case at BCH; we had recently started a Christian memorial service and wanted to offer a wider inclusive provision to all our bereaved families. At this time, we came across the National Memorial Arboretum, near Lichfield in the West Midlands. The beautiful, wide-open nature of the place inspired a couple of us to explore having a memorial there and an annual event. This is now an established part of our bereavement support and we have an annual Walk and Picnic for about 200 family members. We have the riverside sidewalk as our memorial with different size seed-shaped pods at intervals along the walk. Children and young people will be offered an activity before we start our walk, and they will invited to place these things (a windmill, a painted stone with the name of the child they are remembering) at our memorial tree when the adults place a sunflower. There are no prayers, religious blessings, etc. as the aim is to offer pastoral and spiritual care, so everyone feels included.

Rev Paul Nash, chaplain

Patients may be concerned for other family members

Children and young people who are sick may have deep concerns for their siblings, and may not be able to express these easily or to parents. A young person may feel guilty about being the cause of family disruption, where siblings are also suffering loss and separation from parents. Spiritual care activities may well bring these kinds of issues and anxieties to the surface.

PRACTICE EXAMPLE 7.12: ALI'S CRICKET DREAM SPACE

Zamir, the Muslim chaplain, offered the Dream Space activity to 13-year-old Ali. When asked what his dream space was, Ali instantly responded, 'Playing cricket!' He immediately took up paints to create a cricket scene. After giving a few suggestions for use of materials, Zamir wisely withdrew, giving Ali the space, which he evidently needed to concentrate on his artwork and become absorbed in the imaginative exercise.

Returning after about 20 minutes, Zamir discussed his artwork with Ali, seeking to understand and support him. Zamir admired the colourful picture that filled the canvas and noticed that there were no people in the picture. 'Are you in the picture?' she asked of Ali, which is a wonderful open question, important in understanding Ali's sense of identity. Gradually, Ali drew himself, his brother, cousins, his uncle and his mum who was fielding. 'What were the dots around the edges?' Zamir asked. 'That was the crowd of people, watching the game,' Ali replied – so there were people in the picture! At this stage, Ali's mum and dad were in the room with him, and Zamir asked, 'Is Dad in the picture?' Ali replied, 'No.' Clearly something important was being expressed here about the relationship with his Dad. 'Doesn't Dad like to play?' asked Zamir. Rather playfully, Zamir turned to Dad in the room and said, 'Come on, Dad, you need to be in the game as well!'

The moment of awareness and observation seemed significant, made possible through the painting of Ali, and perhaps opening channels of communication which were somewhat closed. Eventually, Dad was also put in the picture as a fielder, but whether that was to appease the situation or express the dream of the child was not certain. Zamir commented that you don't know where you are treading, aware that she had ventured into sacred space with this family, and the tenderness and complexity of their relationships with one another.

Zamir Hussain, chaplain

Summary

Families, and particularly siblings, are on their own spiritual journey and will often welcome any support that can be given:

- Activities with children and young people such as decorating tea lights or making a Hope Blanket square can also engage the parents/carers/siblings and lead to greater understanding and sharing.

- Caring for a child with a disability, temporary or long-lasting, places particular pressures upon families; assessing ability and finding creative approaches will enable every child and young person to be involved.

- Creative approaches to helping families process bereavement and loss can be a significant part of spiritual care.

Chapter 8

Spiritual Practices for Spiritual Care

Introduction

Some of the resources we use for spiritual care are more overtly spiritual. Attending to a child or young person's spiritual identity and offering resources for building them up from the inside will also have an impact on their entire wellbeing. Some of the practices that we have developed relate directly to religious practice, and some can be appropriately used with children and young people with no particular faith background. Part of what is involved in offering spiritual care is offering a vocabulary or means by which spiritual care needs can be communicated. For instance, using colour became a way of one chaplain talking about feelings with a young person who was very quiet and reserved about this kind of conversation. Choosing colours for a beaded bracelet became highly symbolic for the young person who chose yellow beads and then, at a later time, told the chaplain he was having a 'yellow day', a succinct and expressive way of using a shared and newly found language.

Mindfulness

The practice of mindfulness within healthcare is a growing phenomenon rooted in ancient philosophy and religious contemplative traditions. Mindfulness is essentially a moment-to-moment awareness cultivated by paying attention to things we ordinarily do not notice. We are moving from an analytical frame of mind and a place of mental and physical striving into a state of simply being aware of what sensations and feelings are being experienced *at this present moment*. The practice of mindfulness has been shown to have a positive impact on health, wellbeing and happiness (Kabat-Zinn 1990; Williams and Penman 2011). 'The wisdom of our bodies and minds can be used to face stress, pain and illness' (Kabat-Zinn 1990, p.2).

With mindfulness practice, it seems that adults relearn what they knew instinctively as children, particularly as very young children. Children are easily entranced with, and focused on, a particular object, readily experience wonder and awe, and can be caught up easily in the present moment. Some activities help children to become absorbed in a way that offers a relaxing and stilling focus, such as putting stickers in a sticker book, making a bracelet and reflecting on the meaning, or designing patterns and objects using different materials. The simple activity of putting coloured pens back slowly and carefully in a case, noticing each colour in turn and allowing the child to grasp each pen and place them in the case, can be done mindfully. Going at the child's pace will likely slow adults down and bring them into a more mindful awareness, openness and receptiveness to the child. At times, an adult can enable a child or young person to slow down and be centred, which can support peace and relaxation.

Relaxation and visualisation

Children and young people often respond eagerly to gentle practices of stilling the mind using visualisation and the awareness of breathing. If young people have experienced trauma and are having difficulty sleeping or relaxing, mindfulness techniques can aid relaxation and calm them, offering one strategy for managing moments of panic. Learning such techniques empowers children and young people to develop their own resources for self-soothing and support. They do not need to be religious to try these techniques and gain the benefits associated with contemplation, meditation and centring techniques, which strengthen peace of mind. For instance, one young person who was feeling panic and agitation after a traumatic incident was led in a mindfulness exercise, using breathing techniques and the imagination as a strategy for gaining peace on a busy, noisy ward.

PRACTICE EXAMPLE 8.1: WORKING WITH KARA

Kara (12) was feeling anxious and distressed about an upcoming operation on her spine. She was given the suggestion of letting go of anxiety on the out-breath, and on the in-breath imagining a white light flowing into the body. Kara was led in a relaxation exercise, imagining a peaceful, happy place – a holiday destination was chosen – imagining in turn the sights, sounds and sensations of being in that place, as a way of stilling the mind and emotions.

Rev Kathryn Darby, chaplain

Working at the bedside

Awareness exercises at the bedside are possible, although there may be challenges such as frequent interruptions and unexpected noises; however, even practising a few minutes of relaxation can offer young people support in their day and help develop coping strategy for them when the noise and commotion of ward life, constant activity and minimal privacy might be draining. Within their own being, as close as their own breath, there is space and privacy and vast imaginative scope. Craft activities can become a means of quietening the self, bringing the attention into the present moment, and offering rest and strength. One young person volunteered, 'Doing craft activities can help me if I feel worried. They help me to relax.'

Working with groups

Mindfulness and relaxation exercises can be run with groups as well as individuals and can be applicable for a wide age range. Facilitating stilling or centring exercises can help patients connect with their spiritual needs but staff need to be comfortable introducing such activities and feel familiar with imaginative approaches as part of their own practice in order to lead others authentically in such exercises.

ACTIVITY 8.1: RELAXATION AND VISUALISATION EXERCISES

I offered a mindfulness and relaxation exercise in school for a group of ten children made up of in-patients as well as siblings, all part of the primary and secondary classes, ranging in age from 5 to 12 years. The mats were brought out, the tables moved aside and a space cleared for everyone to find a comfortable place on the floor. Some chose to remain seated and it was important to offer this option for those who would struggle to relax on the floor or had disabilities prohibiting this.

For a warm-up exercise, we tried tapping our heads, then rubbing our tummies and, at the same time, closing our eyes and thinking about one thing with one side of our mind, and another with the other side of our mind, and finally, singing a song we all knew together. It was a fun way to discover that our minds can actually do many things at once, but it was also practice in bringing our attention into one place, focusing on the present moment and present awareness in a way that allowed us to relax. Using other exercises, including focusing on our breathing, imagining we were a growing seed, 'watching' our troubles drift above us like a cloud, listening to reflective music, and becoming more aware of how we were feeling in our bodies became further ways of introducing relaxation to the group.

Finally, an imaginative exercise was offered, leading us to picture a happy and peaceful scene of our own making where we entered and spoke with a person who we trusted. These exercises could be shared with children and young people of different faiths or no faith, in order to open up a different kind of space in their day. Asked afterwards what they thought of the session, one child remarked, 'I was bouncing on my bouncy castle!' describing an exhilarating flight of fancy for a young person who had limited mobility at that time.

Rev Kathryn Darby, chaplain

Sometimes it is appropriate for reflection and relaxation time to be offered regularly and can be framed as a spiritual or religious exercise.

ACTIVITY 8.2: MULTISENSORY QUIET TIME

Quiet Time session is a gentle activity offering a number of participants (usually four to six) a quiet space and time for about 45 minutes. The session can be held in a quiet room or quiet open space, or corner of a room, free from as much distraction and noise as possible. It could be held in a quiet corner of the garden on a fine day. Wherever it is held, it should be accessible to staff who may need to come in to tend to any of the children and young people at any given time who may need attention.

An integral part of the session involves the use of an essential oil burning quietly in a safe burner which is lit before the children and young people arrive in the room. I use lemon grass, which over the years has become associated with Quiet Time. A pleasant refreshing aroma pervades the room without it being too overpowering.

In the room, the children and young people usually attend the session sitting in their wheelchairs. There is a small coffee table in the middle of the room, decorated and dressed with a coloured table cloth, or a coloured nylon scarf or a combination of scarfs of different colours that may reflect the colour of the time of year, the seasons, or the liturgical seasons of the year. A battery-powered candle, a fresh flower or a small posy in a vase, one or two significant child-friendly objects add to the integrity of the session. These are placed on the table and are prepared before the session begins.

We gather around the dressed table. I usually sit on a small stool within the circle of wheelchairs near to the CD player with a variety of CDs at hand. I use a number of reflective instrumental musical pieces and/or inspirational or popular songs. A selection of songs and musical pieces are played at intervals throughout the session, usually in sets of three followed by a moment of silence between the sets. The regular intervals of silence are invitations to the sacred to join us. Other times, I begin the session with a guitar instrumental piece that I play myself and end the session with another piece. I then extinguish the candles which is a cue that we are now finished and we leave the room in silence. I record in their medical files they have taken part in the session. This is one example of how I offer a sensory liturgical service to a group of children and young people who live with a multitude of challenges in their lives.

Thomas Begley, hospice chaplain

Religious practice

Within some religious practices, there are signals that help us to realise that we are entering into a holy time and space of prayer or attention to God. For instance, Hindu chaplains will take off their shoes before a time of prayer at the bedside. A Christian chaplain may use a special cloth to set the scene for sharing Holy Communion during a hospital visit. When Mark (4) received his Communion visit, he recognised the special cloth and immediately offered to help the chaplain lay out the cloth and place the items needed for the celebratory meal of bread and wine (non-alcoholic in this context) onto the cloth, making sure that all was ready. The child's knowledge and familiarity with the ritual brought comfort and reassurance, as well as empowerment, as he helped the priest to prepare for the sacramental meal.

PRACTICE EXAMPLE 8.2: DILAN'S STORY
(PART 2) – RELIGIOUS CARE

For some children the most appropriate act of spiritual care is an act of religious care. For example, it was important for Dilan (8), leaving the hospital after a three-month admission, to revisit the intensive care unit in order to lay to rest that experience, which he could not recall. Although Dilan had spent many weeks on the PICU, he had no memory of this critical period in his life, and while he had made an astonishing physical recovery and seemed bright and happy in his waking hours, he was suffering from frightening dreams. We talked together about the idea that just as our physical wounds take time to heal, our spirits also need time to recover from shock and trauma. We planned a visit to the PICU at Dilan's request in order to try to come to terms with what had happened there. Visiting the PICU, we looked at the bed space where Dilan had been (there was no bed in it at that moment). A young girl was sitting up in the neighbouring bed space, and she smiled at Dilan. Several professionals waved at Dilan as he went through the ward, including a nurse who had cared for him, welling up with tears at the sight of his remarkable recovery.

Next, we went to the chapel where I offered Dilan a postcard with a picture of a field of forget-me-not flowers on the front, the word 'Remembering' on the back and a space for a drawing. Dilan drew a picture of himself running from aliens and monsters at high speed and a house on fire. Asking him where he was running to in the dream, Dilan replied, 'I am going to hide behind this tree' as he drew the hiding place into the picture. We talked about the metaphor of 'hiding place' in a religious context (Psalm 34) and talked about the strength of God to help us face anything, God's strength being bigger and stronger than any scary monsters or aliens that might threaten him. 'Remember,' I suggested, 'God is with you always, and not far away; you don't have to run – you just have to turn and God is there.'

In this example, a simple ritual was offered to help heal the wounds of Dilan's spirit. We committed all of Dilan's inner dreams and realities to God as we stood at the altar, said a prayer and sang 'You are my hiding place', while I lay a hand on Dilan's forehead and asked God to continue to heal his spirit. Then Dilan lit a BCH candle. In the chapel was a prayer activity and we looked together in the special golden box, with the question – 'Who does God love?' attached to the box; Dilan lifted the lid and saw a mirror inside and answered, 'The ceiling!' and then, seeing his own reflection, 'Me!' He then wanted to look up biblical verses about God's special love and care for him. Taking the time to participate in a special prayer and ritual for him at this significant time in Dilan's life was a way of taking his needs seriously and emphasising God's love and care for him. Finally, at Dilan's request, we said a prayer for other children in the hospital, and the girl he had seen who was in the PICU, and for his cousin in Sri Lanka who had a fever. Having been self-reflective and made some progress in processing difficult feelings, Dilan's mind turned to concern for other children who were suffering, a recurrent theme in spiritual care with children and young people.

Rev Kathryn Darby, chaplain

Celebrate Religious Festivals project

At BCH we celebrate a wide range of religious and cultural festivals (see Nash *et al.* 2015 for details) and they can be a wonderful opportunity to bring a new point of interest and interaction to children and young people on the wards. Under the banner of the 'Celebrate Project' chaplains at BCH organised simple activities that are taken on to the wards, shared at individual bed spaces, or in small groups on the ward, or in the classroom, including the mental health wards.

Using laminated A4 posters explaining what the festival is about, children are then invited to be creative, making, for instance, at Chinese New Year, paper lanterns and small paper dragon puppets. During the Hindu Holi festival, they might have their face painted or paint a mannequin doll (if face painting was problematic). At Christmas, a Posada idea was developed, based on the Mexican tradition, which involves processing from one house to another carrying the 'holy family' or nativity, the various households acting as 'innkeeper' for one night, which is an opportunity for building community and sharing with one another. Pinatas, traditionally made out of clay, might be broken open to obtain fruit and sweets inside, Christmas carols sung and the story of Christmas recalled. In a similar way, a small trolley was dressed up as a donkey and wheeled on to the wards, filled with Christmas activities and small gifts. Chaplains dressed up as Mary and Joseph and asked the children and young people on the ward if there was a bed free for them for the night – a fun and lively way to bring a new focus into the day and help patients, religious or non-religious, to reflect on the Christmas story and share in the festive spirit. Where possible, involving guests who have experienced these festivals within their own tradition can lend authenticity and vibrancy to the occasion.

A wonderful aspect of the Celebrate Project is the opportunity to inject a little 'normality' into the scenario of being in a hospital together, which is unusual and could even be described as 'not normal'. Children are reminded of the larger world which is still revolving outside of the hospital of which they are a part. Learning about other religions and festivals can enrich life for children and give them a broader perspective during a hospital admission.

ACTIVITY 8.3: EASTER GARDEN

A traditional Christian activity is to create an Easter garden, and one year at BCH we did this in the chapel. Chaplains and youth workers visited children at their bedsides, asking them to paint a stone with a springtime picture on one side of the stone and a message of hope and encouragement for others on the other side of the stone. The children and young people often chose to make two: one to keep and one to share with others. The stones were then brought together to form a path for the garden, and flowers and small clay figures were also shaped holding signs with messages on them.

Visiting one 3-year-old child, Billy, who was not able to use his hands, I drew one of Billy's favourite story characters, Curious George, on the front of the stone checking what colours and ideas would be good for the stone which was left with him. A similar stone featuring Curious George was taken away for the garden. Another older child was shown this stone with the monkey's smiling face and suggested a message for the reverse side: 'Keep going forward swinging from tree to tree'. It was encouraging to take this message back to Billy to share with him and his family. Other stones carried equally joyous and inspiring designs and messages of hope and encouragement: flowers with the accompanying message 'We are all beautiful but delicate'; spiders, chicks, butterflies with the message 'Be beautiful'; a fairy with the message, 'shine'. These all added to a beautiful display that the children could visit and admire in the chapel, and to view their unique contribution which was part of something bigger.

Using metaphors, such as a garden, can strengthen connections that children feel with one another, as well as suggest other layers of meaning – in this case, growth and the beauty and value of each person. Such projects often open doors to important connections for people who are making a significant and sometimes scary and painful journey through the many challenges of being in the hospital. It would be possible to do this activity without the religious location or dimension.

Rev Kathryn Darby, chaplain

Prayer

Prayer may be an integral element of spiritual care and can involve giving an opportunity for children and young people to compose their own prayers. Different resources help facilitate a creative approach to prayer: drawing pictures, using paints and brushes, creating prayer leaves for a tree in the chapel, using Ignatian exercises, such as imagining being in a biblical story and having a conversation with Jesus, or simple prayer ropes, which can prompt a child to think of family, friends and circumstances. Within the Islamic tradition, prayer is believed to be an integral part of daily life, and an act of worship. Through prayer one is acknowledging the power and connection with God. Thus, prayer is not only a very important part of spiritual care, but it also fulfils psychological, emotional, as well as religious needs: 'When my servants ask you (O Muhammad) concerning Me, I am indeed close. I listen to the prayer of every supplicant when he calls on Me' (Quran 2: 186).

Children are usually taught to pray at times of need and distress and to be grateful to God at times of happiness and blessings; also to have forbearance and perseverance at times of difficulties. Thus, dialogue with God is an important part of spiritual care. Many of the activities described above can easily be adapted to use with children and families of different faiths, and are a very useful means of engaging with the child and family to facilitate what can be a healing and meaningful dialogue with God.

After a visit with the chaplain, children and young people may wish to be prayed for. Rather than launching into a prayer based on the chaplain's own perceptions, it is important to ask young people what they would like to pray about or express, opening a window into their own priorities and perspectives.

PRACTICE EXAMPLE 8.3: JOSEFINA'S PRAYER

The chaplain may be surprised by the response a child gives. Despite very serious injuries and a long period of rehabilitation, Josefina didn't pray for herself at all but prayed:

> Thank you Lord for this day that you gave me and thank you for all the children that are laid now in this hospital today. Make them better... Also those going through worse, and for those who's getting out. Thank you Lord for everything you did for them. Make them to thank you. Then show them that you exist. Show them that you are there for them, that you're their Father. Thank you for everything that you did from when I come in till the last day I go away. Thank you, very, very much. Amen.

Being with children and young people encourages us to think of creative ways of praying, using different approaches. For instance, Georgina who was an active member of her church youth group at home, had been involved in a car accident. Georgina had suffered some permanent damage as a result of her accident, including a necessary amputation. Learning to walk again would be slow and difficult and she was anxious about how others might perceive her or bully her, which had been a problem in the past. I offered Georgina a small prayer medallion which held the inscription, 'There is nothing that is going to happen to me today, Lord, that you and I can't handle together.' The inscription on the medallion opened up a conversation about the love and friendship of God, giving strength to overcome obstacles and challenges, taking one step at a time.

ACTIVITY 8.4: IMAGINING GOD

I invite patients to imagine their God sitting down beside them in their room and invite them to share whatever comes to mind with their God. I then ask them if I can write down whatever came to mind and from this we formulate prayers. I ask if we can share the prayers with other people and make up booklets of them which may be helpful for other patients or families. These are some of the prayers; the first one from a teenager, the second one from a 7-year-old:

> *Why does God hate me?*
> *Why does He do the things He does?*
> *Like cancer and problems around the world?*
> *Why did He give me cancer?*
> *He's powerful.*
> *I want Him to take the cancer and make the pain go away.*

> *Dear God,*
> *How do I know how to talk to you*
> *If I've never seen you*
> *And never talked to you before?*
> *I have met other people*
> *But I have never met God.*
> *Why do I have to take medicine?*
> *Why do I have to take a bath?*
> *You are lucky*
> *You don't have to do those things.*
> *But I will have to do them,*
> *So that's why I'm talking to you. Amen.*

Jim Manzardo, chaplain

Prayer may be an integral element in helping children make sense of their experience and it is important to offer opportunities for children to compose their own prayers, using prayer postcards, prayer leaves for a chapel prayer tree, words and letters for composing prayers, prayer beads or bracelets, or mapping and reflection exercises. For children and young people who cannot easily write, a digital recording can be a way to help them express their prayer and understand that it is heard. Given the opportunity, they will often include prayers for other children and young people in the hospital who they have become friendly with, or simply have observed from a distance and see them to be suffering.

Prayer ropes and aids

Chaplaincy has a collection of prayer ropes, each resembling a rosary, but much simpler in design and child-friendly in texture, in a wide range of colours, which are made regularly by a small local church group. Families welcome this colourful prayer rope as a sign of care and in some instances faith and hope. Giving a choice of colours is an important way of making the gift more personal and often the prayer rope will be seen hanging on the bed frame and brightening up the bed space. A prayer rope can be used as a focus of prayer or simply as a reminder and symbol of God's care and connection with that child. Particularly within the Roman Catholic tradition, visual reminders of the faith, such as rosaries, cards with pictures of saints or prayers, and icons may be greatly appreciated.

ACTIVITY 8.5: PRAYER STONES

Within the chapel, a bowl of stones rests on the altar and families are invited to take a stone representing their burden of care and place this on the altar table to be included in the next Holy Communion Service. The prayer stones can be used in different ways according to the instincts of the parent or child. One mum told a chaplain that she had taken the prayer stones and dated them, when God had helped them through a difficult day or a difficult time/procedure, and had built up a small collection of stones, which might then be formed into a piece of artwork or a small cairn.

Other examples include: prayer sticker books and cards (from God Venture), leaves for the prayer tree, prayer bookmarks and postcards. At BCH we have an interactive prayer station within the chapel, which is changed regularly to present different meditations and seasonal focuses for prayer, using pieces of fabric and objects such as interactive prayer cubes, pictures, bowls of coloured pebbles, and other creative means of engaging with God in prayer. One example is a picture of two hands on an A4 laminated sheet, with suggested foci of prayer on each finger. The accompanying text is: 'God holds you in the palm of his hand.' Visitors are invited to reflect prayerfully on these areas of life and then place a 'jewel' (plastic, sticky-backed) on the picture of the hands. Such an exercise can be done in company with family members as they consider together who they are praying for. Although candles cannot remain lit in the chapel due to fire regulations, a simple direction sheet placed in the prayer station prompts families to leave messages and names within candle cases. Candles are then lit for their child at the regular 'Candle Prayers' and the children and young people named are prayed for.

The sense of connection that comes when people understand the needs and situation of the children, and are known to be praying for them, can be very important for a child and their family in hospital, especially when these messages of care come from their school and outside community. We designed Spiritual Care Bandages (see Appendix 2) to build this sense of connection with the wider community. A child is invited to design Spiritual Care Bandages to indicate what is needed for support and also to share with friends and family who can wear these and be reminded of the child in hospital.

ACTIVITY 8.6: RELIGIOUS BRACELETS

Craft suppliers such as Baker Ross in the UK make many seasonal products including bracelets which can be used to tell and explore the story of a particular festival. Visiting children and young people who are religious with materials to make a bracelet telling the Easter story is a simple and enjoyable way to engage with them about the meaning of Easter. Each small square bead has a simple picture on it representing the different stages of Holy Week and as these were carefully strung onto the bracelet, a way was found to engage with a complex story in an accessible and enjoyable way.

As beads were woven together and pause was taken to consider the different parts of the story, a quiet, reflective quality and pace was struck. Questions were asked and conversation shared about the Easter mystery of Christ's death and resurrection. The bracelet was completed and could be worn with pride as others admired the craftwork. As the bracelet was worn, it served as a reminder of the encounter, of meaning, and a possible focus for further reflection. The bracelet that was now being worn by the child was part of his or her story and life experience. Making more of this might be a way to develop the practice, perhaps offering a prayer card that related to the Easter story, reminding the child of the importance and meaning of their faith.

Asking one child, Julia, who she identified with in the story, she replied, 'Mary...because she was brave.' We went on to talk about Mary as a source of inspiration and someone who this child resembled in her courage in the way that she was facing challenges and enduring difficulties. Julia might look at the beads in the future and meditate on the qualities of Mary's existence, building on her own sense of esteem and identity.

Rev Kathryn Darby, chaplain

We recognise that chaplains in particular have a role in nurturing religious faith as an important resource for children and young people who claim this identity. Chaplains can function as experts in their particular faith but are committed to multifaith working (Pattison 2007). For example, Paul was seen in the BBC Two series, *Children's Hospital: The Chaplains*, offering a postcard with suitable words of comfort and encouragement to a Muslim teenager who was just about to go for an operation. In another situation, a member of the child's medical team came to ask us for some resources to offer to a Sikh family, whom she assessed would appreciate some support. She also took more copies of our Sikh prayers for ill children book away, should others ask for it in the future.

Using music and songs

Music and singing can often be therapeutic for children and young people and in some contexts there will be external groups who can support this work.

PRACTICE EXAMPLE 8.4: SINGING MEDICINE

Singing Medicine is a project of the choral group, Ex Cathedra in Birmingham and they come in to BCH weekly and sing with patients believing that hospitalised children and young people should be able to access the arts where they are too. Working with Singing Medicine is a good example of multidisciplinary working, as we can make referrals to them. When we see Singing Medicine with patients, we can tell how much they enjoy listening to and joining in with the singing and we can watch their spirits lift.

You do not need to use religious language but finding songs or making up your own, using the beliefs and desires of the family, is a way of expressing the integrated nature of spiritual care.

How do we offer a soothing presence for a baby or young child who might be upset? Singing to them is a methodology tried and tested over many years and within many cultures. Quiet singing at the bedside can offer a peaceful meditative prayer; often simple settings to blessings can be effective and calming, bringing a personal touch that communicates from one soul to another.

PRACTICE EXAMPLE 8.5: SINGING WITH NEWBORNS

We often sing to neonates and at times hope to offer comfort by making connections with the music they may have heard while still in their mother's womb. I work on the logic that it is not only the words but the tone. When I was a child I always knew by the tone of my mum's voice if I was in trouble or not, there are so many ways in which to say, 'Paul'.

So when I sing quietly, softly, gently, soothingly, 'Peace to you, I bless you now in the name of the Lord, Peace to you. We bless you now in the name of the Prince of Peace, Peace to you' (Graham Kendrick © 1988 Make Way Music), I am seeking to assure the child's inner being, their spirit, that we are speaking good things in their tiny, frail lives, blessing them with Shalom, all the goodness of heaven.

Rev Paul Nash, chaplain

At times, singing can be an effective part of end-of-life prayers. At a baptism service for an infant who was near to death, the song, 'The peace of the earth be with you/the peace of the heavens too/the peace of the rivers be with you/the peace of the oceans too/deep peace falling over you/ God's peace flowing in you...' (Carson and WGRG 1998) was sung and a colleague commented, 'It was like the spirit of God reaching out and surrounding the baby and hovering over the bedside, drawing everyone together and giving a tangible expression to God's presence and holding.' The mother, who had been visibly holding on to her pain and shock with the sudden turn of the baby's health, held her hand to her chest after the blessing was sung, with a small sigh, indicating that she too had been touched and warmed by the song.

PRACTICE EXAMPLE 8.6: BLESSING KATE

Baby Kate was been born at the Women's Hospital and swiftly transferred to the Children's Hospital for urgent surgery to remove a tumour. Her mother was not yet discharged after a difficult labour and her father was also unable to be present at the bedside. I wanted to bridge this gap, offering some gifts of a quilt and a woven cross, as well as visiting and offering a prayer and a sung blessing, offering comfort and reassurance to Kate during a time of upheaval and separation. A blessing, with the warm touch of a hand on her head was a gesture of spiritual care. For babies, the sound of the human voice is known to be connecting and healing.

Rev Kathryn Darby, chaplain

Introducing recorded music can also be a powerful and effective means of bringing comfort and reassurance and a sense of sacredness to significant moments in the life of a family. These songs, contemporary popular tracks or sacred music, can become powerful links for the family, particularly if their child dies. Using John Lennon's (1980) 'Beautiful Boy' for one end-of-life blessing, the grandmother commented much later about how this had become a special song linking her with her grandson.

PRACTICE EXAMPLE 8.7: SINGING WITH WILF

At 9 months, Wilf had physical developmental delay, while his intelligence was noticeably sharp. Very contented in the early days of his admission to hospital, he then experienced some trauma with medical intervention and had developed an appropriate caution around staff as a result. Makaton or British Sign Language can enhance singing, particularly with children who cannot verbalise due to tracheotomies or other conditions.

Bringing a tactile book with appealing images and sharing some singing led to some positive contact and trust building with the chaplain. The book was something he could feel and engage with and he smiled when he turned the pages. Singing a 'Little Bunny' song, at mum's request, brought smiles and pleasure. As the verses were sung, Wilf's little toy bunny was made to touch lightly and dance on his head, the bed, mummy, his hand, etc. Singing the song encouraged him with the clapping that he had just learnt that day. Wilf enjoyed the interaction and moved from being quite still and passive to joining in.

Singing songs and formulating little interactive games – some of the oldest being the best – such as 'the wheels on the bus' – are often warmly received by very young children and their parents. Ideally, chaplains can draw from a memorised repertoire to maximise interaction with the child; but it can also be effective to bring taped music to the bedside and sing along, or bring song books and action books as a guide.

Rev Kathryn Darby, chaplain

Singing to ease anxiety

Music may help to ease anxiety, particularly when singing songs which are familiar to children and young people.

Nadia (9) was on the PICU. Due to a tumour on her spine, she had lost a lot of nerve function, and was essentially paralysed from the neck down, but had some movement and sensations. She was fearful and distressed. Her admission onto the PICU was due to an infection which affected her breathing. As her mum was talking to another professional, the chaplain sat with Nadia, sang some songs from the musical *Joseph* (Lloyd Webber and Rice 1969) and talked about the story of Joseph and fairy stories connected with her doll (Briar Rose Bear). Nadia had so little control in her life, with resulting high levels of frustration, but she was able to say yes by nodding to indicate that she wanted another song and no when she had had enough. She exercised some power through the activity and was able to think about stories and things other than just the interventions of medical staff and her stressful situation, while her mum was freer to unload some of her emotional burden with the visiting psychologist; Nadia was also protected from hearing some of that conversation which might have heightened her anxiety. The following day, Nadia's mum told the chaplain that they had talked some more about the Joseph story after their time together and she had been comforted by the singing.

PRACTICE EXAMPLE 8.8: SOOTHING MARCUS

The chaplain visited Marcus (15 months) who is blind, has delayed learning and had had cranial surgery. Marcus was fractious and the chaplain wondered if, being blind, he had a more acute sense of hearing and might be sensitive to new voices. Some nursery rhymes soothed him – he became still, avidly listening. Marcus picked up a rattle and shook it, responding to the rhythm. His mum was pleased and comforted, saying how Marcus loves to listen to modern pop music on the radio.

Rev Kathryn Darby, chaplain

Singing and music at end of life

On another occasion, the chaplain entered a room where the child had already died and was being held in the arms of her father. It seemed fitting to sing the words of the Gaelic prayer, 'May the road rise up to meet you/May the wind be always at your back/may the sun shine warm upon your face/May the rain fall soft upon your fields/and until we meet again, may God hold you/until we meet again may God hold you/until we meet again may God hold you in the hollow of his hand.' This was sung quietly, kneeling down at eye level with the child, and almost whispering the song to her. Music can express what seem to be inexpressible depths of love, yearning and hope that in the end we will meet again and wholeness will be restored. In order to use songs in this way, a chaplain needs to develop a degree of confidence which can grow, using singing at less significant moments within routine visiting.

Faith stories

There may be occasions when it is important to tell an appropriate story, from the faith tradition or elsewhere, which helps the patient explore meaning. Within the BCH chaplaincy we have developed a range of resources which are faith/religion specific.

Postcards

Postcards with simple messages and pictures can help a child or young person to bring into focus issues they might be dealing with and enable them to communicate about. Building on and connecting with existing spirituality and faith is important. Postcards can offer a non-religious yet spiritual meaning providing comfort, encouragement and hope, with pictures and words that may become a source of meditation. In succinct and profound ways, a verse or statement on a postcard can communicate understanding and reach into the heart of a young person's experience without many words or long explanations. Simply by giving a card that reads, 'Courage doesn't always roar. Sometimes it's the little voice at the end of the day that says I'll try again tomorrow' offers recognition, understanding and hope in the midst of a journey that is fraught and highly charged, yet may be difficult for a child or young person to articulate. Cards can hold a message of peace and hope without diminishing the reality of how challenging and frightening life can be for a child dealing with a serious illness. When postcards offer scope for open and broad reflection they can speak to complex emotional and spiritual journeys while reflecting key principles and sources of hope and inspiration from within a religion. They can also be useful for spiritual care practitioners to offer religious care when this may not be within their tradition but is appropriate for the particular child they are working with.

ACTIVITY 8.7: LABYRINTH POSTCARD

Sally designed a postcard with a labyrinth image on it. The labyrinth has been a tool for reflection and meditation in ancient Roman times and then in Celtic Christian traditions. Unlike a maze which is a complex puzzle with choices of paths and direction, a labyrinth is a single, non-branching path leading to the centre, not designed to be difficult to navigate. While labyrinths are often designed as outdoor circular paths to walk upon, using a finger to trace 'steps' along the postcard labyrinth, children and young people can reflect on their journey: where they have come from, where they are going, what it feels like to be on the path they are on. Often the postcards appear on the wall of a bed space of young people of different faiths and none, indicating that these gifts are of value and worth, reminding young people, too, of the meeting with the spiritual care practitioner who has remembered them and will visit again.

Godly Play

Godly Play (www.godlyplay.uk) is a creative and imaginative approach to Christian nurture and can be used effectively in hospitals, at the bedside or within groups in the hospital school or play room. Using symbols and objects, as well as words and storytelling, Godly Play encourages children to make meaning for themselves and values process, openness and discovery. Listeners are invited into stories and encouraged to connect the stories with personal experience, which can be helpful when a child may be attempting to make sense of difficult and complex experiences. Godly Play also encourages them to move into areas of belief and faith, through wondering questions and open-ended response time. After a story is told, children have the opportunity to interact with the characters in the story, handling the figures and moving them, touching them and speaking to them.

PRACTICE EXAMPLE 8.9: ANNIE AND THE GOOD SHEPHERD

A Godly Play story was taken to Annie (8) who had limited mobility due to a spinal tumour. The story of the Good Shepherd was offered, which is a combination of Psalm 23 and the story of the lost sheep (Luke 15: 1–7). As Annie was lying flat and could not sit up to see the story, the story was told on her bed, which provided some hills for the sheep! First, the visitors and Annie enjoyed imagining what the different bits used to tell the story could be, e.g. green felt might be grass, a blanket or a tablecloth. The chaplain noticed that being imaginative and playful was an effort for Annie. This might have been due to a number of reasons: not being familiar with an approach where 'anything goes' and any meaning is acceptable; possibly reflecting a learnt helplessness where others are creative for her and with her; or perhaps finding it was too much cognitive effort in relation to her illness or medication, recognising that developmental delays can accompany hospitalisation. In any case, Annie's mum was very much involved with the activity, giving many prompts and answers. Perhaps Annie would have contributed more verbally in the absence of the parent; on the other hand, her mum may have given her the confidence to engage in the way she did. Some of Annie's toys on the bed became characters in the story, which brought fun and enjoyment.

The potential resonance of the story with Annie's situation seemed high, with scope to explore themes of identity, safe space, being in danger, being cared for, hope and journey. While using a Christian story, this was done without leading to a religious or churchy discussion. In the wondering/reflection time, Annie's mum nudged her to make many connections with her hospital experience and with her hope of getting out of the current set-up and moving on to better pastures. A section about 'scary places and times' was left open by the chaplain…wondering about when Annie had gone through such times and how she manages to come through while slowly tracing her finger through the dark places. Laughter was shared and trust built, while deeper places were touched upon as well. Providing a visual space, which gave scope for Annie to imagine and move into a different reflective sphere rather than being 'jollied' or 'distracted' by an activity, may well have been the most valuable part of the exercise. Providing a gift or memento of the encounter – a teddy bear with a heart on it – offered further connection and spiritual care.

Rebecca Nye, Godly Play facilitator and Tamsin Cuthbert, children's worker

Working with school groups, it will be important to have some briefing from the teacher beforehand, having some awareness of individual circumstances and taking note of mobility issues, in order to adapt the play/interaction aspect to be as inclusive as possible.

Exploring both the dark and the light

It is important that young people are given scope to explore both the light and dark within the hospital experience, but this needs to be done with sensitivity. Often, adults avoid looking at the negative aspects for fear of making matters worse, but this can lead to greater difficulties for young people who then bury such feelings and questions within themselves or become isolated in their troubles. Processing events in their lives at hospital in this way can be an important part of integrating the sometimes frightening and unsettling experiences of hospital life, placing these aspects, as well as more positive feelings of thanksgiving, joy and celebration into God's care and keeping, where this is part of their worldview.

Need for ritual

Rituals are needed, particularly around death and loss, and even for those who are not religious or do not know what they believe about the afterlife. Sacred moments where loss is acknowledged, private reflections are made, and acts of committing that person in peace and love are an important part of healing and wholeness.

Visiting Todd (17), who was mourning the death of a close friend who had died of cancer, the chaplain learnt that he was unable to attend the funeral due to the fact that he was receiving treatment for cancer himself and was not robust enough to attend. The conversation about his recent loss developed and included a list of other losses and grief. Though not a person of religious faith, there was a need for Todd to find supportive ways to acknowledge his loss, express his pain, and connect with the reality that his friend had died. He gladly received the offered prayer rope which he held on to tightly, symbolising in some way the life of his friend, and he held the chaplain's hand while she prayed that Todd would find strength to let go of those who had died and to be assured they are free and to embrace his life, fulfil his dreams and be blessed. At the end, he cried gentle tears and spoke of his own sense of inadequacy with prayer: what should he say? The chaplain suggested that it is not about being eloquent but about being real. Todd placed the prayer rope in a privileged position – around the neck of a special teddy that had been his companion throughout his seven years of cancer treatment, thus signifying the significance of what it now represented. Following on from this experience, Todd discovered the chapel for the first time, and cheerfully requesting several more prayer ropes of different and varied colours to give to friends and family; he also gave the chaplain a donation for the chapel.

ACTIVITY 8.8: GOLD HEARTS

One of the most frequently used resources at BCH is our gold hearts. They are small padded hearts and can be used by any member of staff. When a family request prayers or a blessing for their child, they are offered the hearts as a way of them taking part. We place a dish of the hearts on the child's bed and invite those present to come individually and lay a heart on or around the child as a sign and symbol of their love for them and to take one away to represent the love that the child has for them. When all those who want to take part have done so, I invite the family to lay a heart on behalf of those who love the child and cannot be with them at this time. I invite the nurse to come and place one to represent the care of the hospital and I come and lay one as a sign of God's love for them. The reason why this activity is so popular is that it requires no words, anyone can take part.

I recently offered this to a family who were struggling with the sudden, pending operation of their sedated young child on Christmas Eve, and it was seen as a loving, giving and receiving gift. I offered two small gold bags, one for the family to keep safe those hearts for other members of the family, and another for the nurse to keep the patient's heart together and safe when the bedding is changed or procedures need to be done.

Rev Paul Nash, chaplain

Tea lights

Lighting candles is a feature of all world religions and can be a significant symbol for finding strength, courage, hope and inspiration in the midst of darkness. Taking this powerful yet simple symbol to children in the form of tea lights to decorate and customise has been an effective spiritual care tool. Although candles cannot be lit in the hospital, a battery-operated candle provides a fun alternative. While painting the glass tea light holder, young people can reflect with the spiritual care practitioner on sources of hope and courage, choosing colours and designs that represent their favourite things. Visiting Jemma at home during the palliative phase of her life, these candle holders made with the chaplain while she was in hospital were lit for each member of her family and kept within sight, representing the family unity and love alongside her, and also the strength of light over darkness.

PRACTICE EXAMPLE 8.10: BRIAR TINKERBELL
AND A LIGHT FOR NANNY

A routine visit on the neurological ward led to a 'chance' encounter with Briar (5) who I had met several years previously. At birth, there were health complications for Briar, which led to over a year in hospital, and our relationship had been built then. Briar is profoundly deaf and has significant sight impairment but communicates fluently in British Sign Language with her mum who is a qualified teacher of British Sign Language. In addition to the upheaval of being in hospital for a cranial procedure, Briar's grandmother had died only three days previously and it was Briar who had discovered her body. Briar's brother, Flint (4), had also been highly disturbed by the sudden death of his grandmother and had become extremely anxious about Briar's hospital admission. Briar's mum was having to manage her own feelings of shock and grief at the loss of her mother while supporting her two children through their distress and loss and Briar through an operation.

After speaking with Briar and her mum about their experience of loss, I made several suggestions for helping to process and contain their shock and grief. Briar decorated a glass tea light holder and prepared prayers on leaves for the prayer tree in the chapel. Briar wrote 'Nanny' on the side of her tea light and was pleased with the battery-operated 'candle' and the idea that she was doing something special for her grandma. The idea that 'Grandma's light had gone out on earth but gone on in heaven' was spoken by Briar's mum with the wonderfully descriptive sign language of hands opening and moving towards the sky. A quiet moment was shared as Briar 'lit' her flame and watched her mother translate my prayer for Briar, her grandmother and all the family. In such ways, children can be supported in beginning to make sense of loss and find peace in troubling situations.

Rev Kathryn Darby, chaplain

Visiting within mental health

Young people with mental health issues – depression, experiencing visual or auditory hallucinations, self-harming or eating disorders – need the support of adults to find their way through an often frightening and disorientating period of life. Questions and concerns of a religious or spiritual nature may arise. Adolescents who have self-harmed may be concerned about their relationship with God and may be asking if God will punish them because of what they have done. 'People with psychotic depression can exaggerate religious guilt to a delusional degree' (Griffith 2012, p.231). There may be a place within mental health for the element of confession and absolution, enabling a degree of self-acceptance which might not be achievable within the realm of psychological therapies alone. If a young person would like prayers said, it is important to ask them what they would like to say to God in order to be truly reflective of their desire before God.

Within acute care, staff who are primarily accustomed to nursing children and young people suffering with natural illnesses can struggle when caring for young people who have caused themselves harm; staff may even give conscious or unconscious signals of judgement and disapproval. Disappointment and judgement may also be communicated by family members, along with the anxiety and desire for their recovery. The chaplain may be able to address the balance of silent reproof by offering acceptance, warmth and genuine positive regard. Offering the young person the opportunity to express in some way their sense of guilt, and taking this seriously by listening carefully and offering a prayer of acceptance might give some relief. Using the visual prompt of the Examen doll can be a way of reflecting on the happy and sad or confused parts of ourselves which can all be brought before God in a prayer, exploring what is difficult and asking God's help if appropriate, or noticing what has been uplifting in the day and offering gratitude. There is research to suggest that mindfulness practice can offer support and relief for those suffering with depression and anxiety.

Human love and kindness

The underpinning common strand in effective spiritual care is about one person caring enough to reach out to another person and being open to the gifts and graces that will meet them in that encounter. A sense of hope and relatedness nourishes the spirit, gives strength and can link with a person's will to live (Narayanasamy 2010, p.49). Caring people are at the heart of spiritual care and that is something that every staff member can aspire to be.

Our research with young people with cancer bore this assertion out. Investigating what gave resilience to young people with cancer, the question was asked, 'What gave you strength? What kept your spirits up?' and the answers often included the presence and support of others, family, friends, but also staff. One young person talked about the nurse who came beside her and held her hand and stroked her arm and said, 'When you need me, I will come and sit with you.' Another liked it when the chaplain held her hand and said a prayer for her. Small acts of kindness speak volumes for a child or young person in hospital. Taking the trouble to remember the wishes and requests of a young person can be immensely supportive at a time when they are feeling vulnerable: 'It's nice,' said Laura, 'when they think about me.' When celebrating the Chinese New Year, a volunteer called Tjutju, originally from Singapore, was invited to join in the festivities in order to share her experience and knowledge about the festival. One child who had been in the hospital for several months was excited about Tjutju's upcoming visit and greeted her with energy and enthusiasm, 'Are you Tjutju?' The name 'Tjutju' means 'the first light of the dawn', our friend explained, although, she added, 'In Britain, it means 'the sound of a train!' Her visit with the young people signalled in some measure the light of the dawn, the hope that rises in our hearts when we meet with another person who cares enough to bother. The real human contact that can be offered in straightforward meetings and in more creative, innovative ways is the true substance of spiritual care.

PRACTICE EXAMPLE 8.11: JOSEFINA'S STORY

Josefina was 14 when she was first admitted at BCH (see also Practice Example 8.3). Having suffered extensive burns in a house fire, she received intensive care treatment for several months before moving onto the burns unit for further treatment and rehabilitation. We met Josefina in the early days and began to learn of her story. Many professionals formed a strong team devoted to her care, bringing a wide range of expertise and compassion.

Knowing her to be part of a Christian family, chaplaincy also began regular contact with Josefina, offering visits and prayers. At this stage, Josefina was only beginning to gain consciousness and a tracheotomy meant that she could not speak or communicate easily. The news of her father's death came necessarily after his funeral had taken place, and it was difficult to imagine Josefina's pain and heartache, now an orphan, as her mother had died years ago, but supported by her loving group of sisters and extended family. Josefina appreciated the support of her growing hospital family. When she was ready, one of the chaplains helped to organise a memorial service for Josefina's father, which was held in the hospital, and by this point Josefina was able to leave the burns unit in a wheelchair, to sit at the front of the chapel and at her place in the heart of her family.

Towards the end of Josefina's 18-month stay we looked at the card 'Teddy's in hospital' (with a picture of a Teddy with a bandaged head and arm in a sling), which allows the patient to talk vicariously. This is part of the transcript:

> *K:* (Chaplain) So you're saying…Teddy will feel scared, he might be feeling pain, and he's scared about…what will happen to him maybe…

> *J:* Yeah, he doesn't know what's gonna happen to his arm or to his head (yeah). He might think that he'll never be able to move them 'cause they're like in bandages (um).

> *K:* And would it help if someone explained?

> *J:* Yeah! I think it would help if like the nurses explained to him what's gonna happen, that it's gonna be okay, (um) that later or soon he's gonna be able to move his arms and his legs, run around and jump, and he'll have no problem with that.

K: So they explain what's going on. It must be very bewildering if he's thinking in his head…

J: If the nurse tells him what's gonna happen soon he might be relieved, he might be thinkin', oh, I'm not gonna be able to move it now cause the nurses told him what's gonna happen; he might be saying, okay, so I'm not gonna worry about it no more 'cause I might be able to move it later. I'm gonna be okay, the nurse and the doctor are around me.

K: Is there anything else Teddy might be scared about?

J: That some people might treat him different – just 'cause he's got a broken arm and bandages on his head.

K: Hm…he just wants to be treated the same as everyone else.

I went on to talk about the importance for Josefina of her faith, her music and singing in church. Josefina expressed her values and insight: communicating clearly with children about their situation to help alleviate fears, the importance of small gifts and signs of love from the community, enjoying favourite foods, developing positive relationships within the hospital community, having people to talk to and share with, being encouraged in order to build resilience and hope for the future. Josefina, who had endured great loss and physical changes, receiving several amputations and numerous skin grafts and treatments, suggests that Teddy 'just wants to be treated the same as everyone else'. Her responses were echoed in our research with young people with cancer who identified similar priorities and the desire to 'get back to normal'.

While life can never return exactly to where it was, a new normal can be found, and children can be supported in developing a strong and healthy identity, taking their place in the world. With the love of her family and the support of a dedicated staff team, including a play specialist on the burns unit, physiotherapists, surgeons, nurses and chaplains, Josefina walked out of the hospital to new challenges and also public recognition for her bravery.

Rev Kathryn Darby, chaplain

Summary

- Exercises in mindfulness, relaxation and visualisation can help to ease anxiety, develop coping strategies for and support the spirit of children and young people.

- Music can be used to soothe, stimulate, engage with patients.

- At times spiritual care is deepened with religious care, which may include inspiring texts and postcards, faith stories, prayers and simple rituals.

- The most valuable tool is being a loving, compassionate person who treats the patient with care and respect and leaves behind a sense of that positive regard.

- Reciprocity is important – the professional is also on a journey of spiritual growth and discovery and will be enriched by the encounters with others.

- The personal spirituality and faith tradition (if any) of the spiritual care practitioner may influence the type and extent to which they engage in spiritual practices with others.

Chapter 9

Tensions and Issues

Sometimes spiritual care may seem to be a bit of a nebulous concept and much harder to identify than physical or medical care, for example. However, if we ignore a child or young person's spirituality we may not achieve the best care outcomes:

> For a human being, especially a child or young person, to have a full quality of life, spirituality in all its aspects must be nurtured and affirmed. For children or young people who have been marginalised or who have suffered deprivation in every way, the need for such nurture and affirmation in human spirituality is all the more pronounced. (Bradford 1995, p.2)

A significant tension may be different perspectives on what spiritual care is and what the role of various staff and volunteers may be within it. There is also the issue of when spiritual care blends into religious care and while some may be happy offering the former they do not want to or feel ill-equipped to do the latter.

Whose job is spiritual care?

Because there is still a tendency to equate spiritual with religious, there can be some reluctance to engage with spiritual care and many see it as the responsibility of the religious care specialists, despite the widespread research and literature about spiritual care for all sorts of professionals working with children and young people. It is important to realise that spiritual care happens within a community and through the life of a community, as well as one-to-one. The wider issues of what a child or young person picks up about who they are, their value in the world, their identity and so on all impact them (whether they are aware of it or not) which means that it is important that the whole community caring for them takes responsibility for this dimension of spiritual care.

Motivation

One of the issues around offering spiritual care may be our motivation for doing so. This list of motives may help you explore your own practice:

- It's part of my job.
- It's the most exciting part of what I do.
- It's a box I have to tick.
- I enjoy listening to people and helping them explore their thoughts and experiences.
- I like to see children and young people growing and developing.
- My own experience helps me to see how valuable it is.
- I enjoy caring for the whole person.
- I'd feel more confident if I understood more about the whys and hows.

Some of these comments may trigger thoughts which can usefully be discussed in supervision or as part of a reflective practice activity or just to think through a bit further.

Self-awareness

In some ways, the more we are aware of and comfortable with our own spirituality the easier it may be to engage with others over theirs. As discussed previously, Csinos and Bellous (2009) identify four spiritual styles and being aware of what our own preferences are, but also how others may engage with spirituality, can help in our approach to spiritual care. The four are:

- word-centred – the path of the intellect
- emotion-centred – the way of the emotions
- symbol-centred – the journey of mystery
- action-centred – the road to justice.

As with all such models, they are useful in giving insight to a topic, but are not the only approach, and we may have a spirituality that combines different elements of each. What is helpful with this model is it can help us to reflect as we design spiritual care activities and to consider different dimensions of spirituality, particularly when we work with groups.

Many of us will be aware of communication theory, which suggests that our words account for only 7 per cent of what is received (verbal), tone, pitch and volume is 38 per cent (paraverbal), and body language and behaviour 55 per cent (non-verbal) (O'Connell 2013, pp.59–60). Thus, we need to reflect on what we are communicating when we engage in spiritual care and if we are not comfortable, then we may well communicate that to the children and young people we are working with. Our underlying mood may also come across and we need to be conscious of our speech patterns and non-verbal behaviour and try to ensure that they are consistent. For example, if you are telling someone you are not cross or annoyed with them but have a stern face and harsh voice, they are more likely to trust what they see than what they hear. Conversely, when you say, 'That was a cheeky thing to do,' but you are smiling and your tone is light, usually children and young people will see that you are being light-hearted with them. We also need to know how to interpret the way that others are communicating with us and be aware of any cultural preferences, practices or organisational guidelines which set boundaries in our encounters with children and young people.

Communicating about ourselves

One of the tensions with spiritual care may be what we disclose about ourselves and what the role of that might be in building positive relationships.

PRACTICE EXAMPLE 9.1: LILLY'S OPERATION

Lilly (10): I've never had a big operation before…

Chaplain: How are you feeling about the operation?

Lilly: I don't know.

Chaplain: As you say, it's all new for you.

Lilly: Yeah, and I guess I feel scared about it.

Chaplain: Sometimes when I feel scared, my tummy feels funny.

Lilly: Me too. My mum said I don't need to feel scared.

Chaplain: Sometimes we just do…that's okay. It's okay to feel scared sometimes. But there will be lots of people to look after you. And your mum will be here too. Everyone will care for you.

Disclosing something about myself helped develop a conversation about the child being scared. However, we need to be careful not to over-share and cause discomfort to a child or young person.

Rev Kathryn Darby, chaplain

There are some things we should avoid when thinking about what we share with others:

- Implying that we fully understand someone's situation because we have had a similar experience.

- Burdening others with our own problems.

- Confusing being friendly with being friends.

- Turning the focus of the conversation onto ourselves and our own situation rather than staying focused on the child or young person.

- Doing more talking then listening leading to others feeling undervalued in the conversation.

- Disclosing more to some than others could suggest you have favourites.

- Not feeling comfortable with silence so filling it with our own stories rather than giving others thinking time.

(Petrie 2011, pp.84–89)

This is a helpful list to reflect on and consider in the light of our professional practice, remembering how complex it can be sometimes to separate personal and professional selves.

PRACTICE EXAMPLE 9.2: TO SHARE OR NOT TO SHARE?

One of the chaplaincy team at BCH, Rachel Hill-Brown, has a daughter with Down syndrome and she observes that having a child with a disability has changed her and given her some experiences in common with the families she works with. She comments that, 'Whether or not I choose to share this information with those families is a decision I always take with care but I have always done my best to ensure that sharing my story will be helpful for the family I support rather than some kind of cathartic experience for me.'

Rachel has also found that colleagues refer her to families who also have a child with Down syndrome and she recalls how 'a unique place emerges where shared experience opens the way to support and hope. My colleagues have clearly observed this space when they have encountered parents of mostly babies with Down syndrome. At a point where shock, grief, fear and loss are the world where patients find themselves, chaplains do their best to listen, to comfort, to be present and to pray and if they have a colleague who shares some aspect of the family's story, they make the local connection and an informal referral takes place. This has the potential to be a catalyst for change, change for the better.'

However, there are some tensions inherent in such a practice and the UK Board of Healthcare Chaplaincy refers to practising ethically in capability 3, which involves non-maleficence, doing no harm; beneficence, seeking well-being and respect for autonomy and justice (UK Board of Healthcare Chaplaincy 2014).

Rachel reflects, 'Using these reference points in relation to my experience here it is clear that whether it is myself personally, or someone acting on my behalf, that a desire to do no harm and to seek the well being of the whole family is paramount. Questions of autonomy and justice are also relevant here. Data protection and confidentiality mean that patients and their stories are held in confidence and are only shared with permission or for essential professional reasons (safeguarding). If a patient or parent chooses to disclose an aspect of their story with a chaplain, it remains our responsibility to treat it with confidentiality. This also includes the stories belonging to the chaplains themselves. In just the same way as we do not discuss patients and their families with other patients and families we should not discuss the stories owned by chaplains. And yet, we do tell aspects of our own stories and even, whilst being careful to protect their identity, tell stories of other families who have trod this way before. Our intention is always to encourage, show compassion and understanding and to give some sense of hope, which might make the road travelled seem less lonely. But I also have the responsibility to protect my daughter and not to take advantage of her for my direct benefit or even for others whom I support. There is a balance to be sought and constantly reviewed.'

Such reflections can be applied to a variety of other issues and being reflective of our own spiritual care practice is vital if we are to practice ethically.

Empowerment

Empowerment is a core underpinning value of spiritual care, which is not something we impose on children and young people. Empowerment is about helping them to understand, respond to and act upon the things which are important to them and their wider community. Empowerment is about dialoguing together about what the options may be and encouraging young people to identify responses to their difficulties and dilemmas, rather than just offering them solutions or answers ourselves. At the very simplest level it is about allowing young people to make the decision as to whether or not to engage with us in the first place. Then, it may be about what sort of shared activity or experience we engage with and also about what they do about the issues raised. In some contexts this may not be what children are used to and it can take some time to help them to function in an empowered way. In hospitals, for example, much of what happens there is (rightly) no choice, and it may take a bit of a switch of mindset for them to develop the autonomy to make choices relating to spiritual care. A particular tension is working out how strongly to encourage a reluctant child to take part in an activity, as ultimately it may be in their best interest to do so. Another tension is the balance between the wishes of young people and those of their families.

PRACTICE EXAMPLE 9.3: EMPOWERING YOUNAS

The chaplain knocked and entered a cubicle where Younas (10) was watching *Batman* on his TV. The chaplain was conscious of the fact that Younas might resent being disturbed whilst watching the film, so she introduced herself and asked if it would be okay for her to stay, or should she come back another time. Having gained permission, she offered Younas a choice of Islamic scratch bookmarkers, which he took and started to work on after some prompting. She tried to engage him in some conversation but finding this was not flowing very easily decided that this was enough for the first encounter. She asked if he would like her to go so that he could carry on watching the film and he said 'yes'. She had told him the days she worked and asked him if it would be okay to come and see him again. He shrugged his shoulders but as she opened the door to leave, he said, 'Will you come back to see me on Thursday?'

Zamir Hussain, chaplain

Referrals

Another tension is knowing when to make a referral. In spiritual care it is important that we are aware of our own experience and limitations and make referrals to appropriate others where an issue falls outside our own expertise. Thus, sometimes when patients want to talk about their faith as part of spiritual care a referral will be made to a chaplain who is an expert in this area. On another occasion, a chaplain was talking to a parent who was sharing how difficult it was to find the fares to keep on visiting and, with their permission, the parent was referred to the ward social worker. What is particularly important is the way we negotiate a referral as we need to avoid the child feeling rejected or brushed off. Where children have the capacity to do this, then we should try to help them share the ownership of the decision and understand why it is happening. Some of the questions we may want to ask ourselves about a particular situation include:

- Do I have the necessary experience?
- Do I have sufficient knowledge?
- How does this fit in with my job description/role?
- Do I have the necessary resources (time, emotional energy, etc.)?

- Is it appropriate?

- What practical implications are there?

- Do I need to check this out first?

- Are others more suitable/better equipped?

We also need to be aware that sometimes people will not take up the opportunity a referral offers for various reasons and anything we can do to facilitate this will be helpful.

Resources

The following activities are resources we use as tools for reflective practice, either ourselves or with staff or patients. They help explore some of the tensions and issues that may be present in a particular situation. There are also many good books with useful exercises which can be adapted for spiritual care (e.g. Darley and Heath 2008; Liebmann 2004; Malchiodi 1998; Sunderland and Engleheart 1993).

ACTIVITY 9.1: THE WINDOW

Take a picture of a four-paned window and identify four different areas to reflect on, for example, past, present, preferred future and feared future. Another option would be hopes, dreams, fears, changes. In essence, it could be used for any reflection where we want to look at four elements.

ACTIVITY 9.2: MANDALAS

Mandalas have been used for centuries for spiritual enlightenment across a range of religious traditions. A mandala is an image which is created within a circle, often with a range of colours. The circle can be any size, although some think that 10" diameter is good, about the size of a dinner plate. Others consider a circle within a square is good, as Jung suggested that this was a representation of self. Oil pastels work well for this but choose any media you like; sometimes mixed media is effective, as texture, as well as colour, can be significant.

- Draw a circle on the chosen piece of paper.

- The circle can be filled in however you like, using any media you like. It doesn't matter where you start, whether it is geometric or not, nor if you go outside of the circle. There is no right or wrong way to draw it. But for future reference it can be useful to make it clear which way up it goes. Putting in a place and a date may help evoke the wider memories associated with it.

- Displaying the mandala can help to get the most out of our 'reflection' and sometimes we see something we didn't realise first time round.

ACTIVITY 9.3: METAPHORICAL PORTRAITS

Many of us will have played games at parties where we have to answer a question, such as if you were an animal what sort of animal would you like to be? This idea can be adapted to use with many art media and can cover so many different triggers such as: house, food, tree, flower, island, building, plant, landscape, car, bird, game, place and, where appropriate, add a context. We may then reflect on what we chose and why. Liebmann (2004, pp.228–9) suggests some helpful questions which help facilitate reflection on the portrait, including:

- What object would you like to be?

- What object represents how you feel today?

- What animal, etc. would you most or least like to be?

- If you were a seed what point of growth would you be at?

ACTIVITY 9.4: VOMIT BOWL AND LOCKER

Encouraging the identification and naming of difficult experiences and emotions is a helpful dimension of spiritual care. Sometimes it can be helpful to do an exercise where we encourage children and young people or others to do something metaphorically with these feelings. A physical or drawn vomit bowl can be used to put in those things we want to discard and, it is hoped, never see again by writing or drawing, as appropriate. Where there are emotions or experiences that we are aware of but are not ready to process, we can then write them into a picture of a locker or on scraps of paper to put into the locker (or substitute, such as a small box).

Self-care

As a chaplaincy team we offer self-care sessions to various teams across the hospital, as well as to newly qualified nurses. In the first session we nearly always give out a card which has these words on it: 'Self care is never a selfish act – it is simply good stewardship of the only gift I have, the gift I was put on earth to offer others. Anytime we can listen to our true self and give it the care it requires, we do it not only for ourselves, but for the many others whose lives we touch' (Palmer 1999, p.30).

PRACTICE EXAMPLE 9.4: ACTIVITIES THAT
PROMOTE WELLBEING AND SELF-CARE

In an empirical research project (Nash 2011) among caring professions, including healthcare, I found a range of practices which enhance self-care and wellbeing:

- Care equally for ourselves and those close to us as we do for patients.

- Good quality continuing professional development.

- Ensure proper time off and good work–life balance.

- Make time for self in windows during the day.

- Celebrate achievement or other significant milestones including personal ones.

- Note positive feedback from managers, colleagues, patients and experts.

- External support – formally, non-clinical supervision, mentoring, coaching, etc. and informally, having someone you can offload to.

- Process negative emotions – deal with disappointment proactively and talk things through, don't bottle them up.

- Express gratitude and appreciation.

- Be willing to question, reassess, realise that change means change of pattern.

Rev Dr Sally Nash, chaplaincy researcher

Thus, as spiritual care practitioners we need to pay attention to our own spiritual resources and ensure that when we have been involved in situations which have depleted us we find ways of replenishing ourselves. That may mean five minutes to listen to a favourite song, a brief brisk walk or some silence in chapel to begin to pay attention to our own needs.

PRACTICE EXAMPLE 9.5: STAFF SUPPORT

One of the interesting consequences of doing this kind of work with the patients is that staff have made the connection with their own spiritual needs. One lovely story is when we were exploring staff self-care around resilience and wellbeing, with some of our Emergency Department team. I told a story of the examen lolly stick people activity and what made the children and young people both sad and happy. One nurse piped up and said that she played this game at university. The group asked her to explain and she told us that she and her friend would play the high-low game at the end of each day of lectures. With the high-low game you go round the circle and each of you shares a high point and low point of the shift or week, for example. The rest of the staff team were really taken aback by the helpfulness of this exercise. They suggested that they use it to process what has happened during their shifts and help them gain perspective on both the high and the low points. This would enable them to leave some of the less helpful aspects at work and not take them home.

Rev Paul Nash, chaplain

It may also be important to be involved in corporate, as well as individual, self-care and make the most of the resources available within our organisation and formal and informal networks.

ACTIVITY 9.5: PELICAN CARD

We have a card with a picture of a pelican plucking its own breast. Legend has it that they do this to feed their young if no other food is available. On the card are the words 'caring sometimes hurts'. We use it as a starting point in staff debriefing meetings, or even with families, to explore some of the issues they are facing.

Prayer

For multidisciplinary staff, as opposed to chaplains, prayer may become an issue. In the UK, there have been instances of healthcare staff being disciplined for inappropriately offering to pray for patients, yet our definition of spiritual care involves the potential for a relationship with the transcendent or God. It is very important to understand the boundaries and professional practice guidelines in our own setting and to be clear as to what it means to get voluntary informed consent for anything which may be perceived as outside of normal treatment or care.

On the wards

There are around 350 patients staying in BCH at any one time, and while not everyone wants a visit from a chaplain or spiritual care practitioner, there are tensions as to how one prioritises one's time and the balance between long-term relationships with long-stay patients and meeting one-off needs. It can be very difficult visiting one child with something special to do and seeing their neighbours looking on longingly, possibly wondering when it is their turn for a visit. But for our interpretive spiritual encounters to work, we do need to give a reasonable amount of time to a particular child to be able to make an assessment which leads to further interventions and a spiritual care plan.

While there are well over 40 ideas in this book, if you imagine a long-term patient that you see a couple of times a week, it is difficult to always have something new and inventive to offer. In those circumstances, trying to have some activities that can be recurring may be useful. The examen doll is relevant for any meeting and it may be helpful to encourage young people to reflect on any recurring patterns that make them choose the happy face or the sad one.

ACTIVITY 9.6: WHAT'S THE WEATHER LIKE TODAY?

We have talked about finding simple ways of expressing the more complex things that children and young people may be experiencing. Encouraging them to draw their own weather chart and symbols and to record them regularly can be a way of seeing how they are doing. Again, it may be something you would want to ask open-ended questions about, and also to encourage a full range of symbols which may help them to distinguish between a typhoon and heavy rain! Daily weather charts may encourage children, if they see that storms are happening less frequently, for example. It is also something which could be done with a family together and may offer a language to discuss emotion.

Summary

- Understanding what motivates us to do spiritual care is important along with understanding our own spirituality.

- It is important to think through our own experiences and when, and if, we should share them for the benefit for those we are working with.

- Referrals should be made as appropriate while assuring children and young people of our ongoing concern for them.

- Self-care is vital if we are to be effective spiritual care practitioners.

Chapter 10

Facilitating Spiritual Literacy

At the beginning of this chapter, you may like to reflect on some questions to help you think about your own spiritual journey; you may even want to do this exercise with others you work with at some point.

ACTIVITY 10.1: EXPLORING OUR OWN SPIRITUAL JOURNEY

Using a sheet of paper divided into four, use each quarter to write or draw:

- something you are passionate about

- something that lifts your spirits

- a person who has been influential in your spiritual or life journey

- a place that is sacred or special to you in some way.

You could make up your own questions or even play spiritual experience bingo. Spiritual experience bingo is where you have a grid with say 20 spaces on it, each one having a spiritual experience in it, such as climbed a mountain, saw a rainbow, meditated in the last week, attended a religious service and you have to meet someone in the room who has had that spiritual experience. First one to complete the card wins. in a room where you have a list of things and you need to find someone who has done each one. These could range from making a snow angel to attending a worship service at festival time or giving to a charity. These sorts of exercises help us to understand how broad the activities and experiences are which may be regarded as spiritual. We often say that spiritual care is more easily caught than taught, but when we begin to talk about facilitating spiritual literacy we may find it helpful to offer a variety of lenses that allow spiritual-care practitioners to understand more about the broader context they are working within. The following models are some that we find helpful in conceptualising some of the work that we do.

Fisher's four domains of spiritual health and wellbeing

Fisher (2011) explores the idea of spiritual health and wellbeing, which he sees as having four domains that relate to the relationship someone has with themselves, with others, with nature/their environment and with the transcendent and/or God. The quality of relationships in these domains influences someone's spiritual health and wellbeing and is relevant to all types of belief from strong atheist to committed deist. His model is summarised in Table 10.1. Knowledge (the first row) is the cognitive framework which interprets the inspirational element (or 'head and heart', second row) and the third row shows how this domain may be expressed in life. A greater positive engagement with these domains improves spiritual health.

Underpinning this model is Fisher's definition of spirituality:

Spirituality is concerned with a person's awareness of the existence and experience of inner feelings and beliefs, which give purpose, meaning and value to life. Spirituality helps individuals to live at peace with themselves, to love (God and) their neighbour, and to live in harmony with the environment. For some, spirituality involves an encounter with God, or transcendent reality, which can occur in or out of the context of organized religion, whereas for others, it involves no experience or belief in the supernatural. (2011, p.20)

Fisher's work can be useful in identifying ways in which to engage children and young people that will enhance their spiritual health. It also enables spiritual care to be delivered with a particular focus if, for example, one identifies a domain where further work is particularly significant.

TABLE 10.1: FOUR DOMAINS OF SPIRITUAL HEALTH AND WELLBEING

Domain / Factors	Personal	Communal	Environmental	Transcendental
Knowledge aspect: • filtered by world view	Meaning, purpose and values	Morality, culture (and religion)	Care, nurture and stewardship of the physical, eco-political and social environment	Transcendent other: • ultimate concern • cosmic force, New Age • God, for theists
Inspirational aspect: • essence and motivation • filtered by beliefs	Human spirit creates awareness, self-consciousness	In-depth interpersonal relations reaching the heart of humanity	Connectedness with nature/creation	Faith
Expressed as	Joy, fulfilment, peace, patience, freedom, humility, identity, integrity, creativity, intuition, self-worth	Love, forgiveness, justice, hope and faith in humanity, trust	Sense of awe and wonder, valuing nature/creation	Adoration and worship being: • at one with Creator • of the essence of the universe • in tune with God

Source: adapted from Fisher 2011, p.23

McSherry and Cash's taxonomy of spirituality

Drawing on a literature review, McSherry and Cash (2004) have developed a taxonomy of spirituality that, while it has acknowledged limitations, demonstrates the breadth of definitions that are to be found in the healthcare literature. It may be helpful to locate our own and others' understandings within such a framework, as that might help us to identify possible disparities in approach, and encourage us to develop some shared vocabulary and understandings to ensure that when spirituality and spiritual care is discussed there are some commonalities.

TABLE 10.2: A TAXONOMY OF SPIRITUALITY

Theistic	Belief in a supreme being, cosmological arguments not necessarily a 'God' but deity
Religious	Affiliation – belief in a God, undertaking certain religious practices, customs and rituals
Language	Individuals may use certain language when defining spirituality such as inner strength, inner peace
Cultural, political, social ideologies	An individual may subscribe to a particular political position or social ideology that influences/governs their attitudes and behaviours dependent upon world faith – religious tenets
Phenomenological	One learns about life by living and learning from a variety of situations and experience, both positive and negative
Existential	A semantic philosophy of life and being, finding meaning, purpose and fulfilment in all of life's events
Quality of life	Although quality of life is not explicit in definitions, it is implicit
Mystical	Relationship between the transcendent, interpersonal, transpersonal, life after death

Source: adapted from McSherry and Cash 2004, p.155

Quaker spirituality model

The Quaker model encourages a focus on upward, inward, outward and downward, thus offering a different four domains to reflect on in our spiritual care. It resonates with some of our research findings and can be used regardless of a presence or absence of religious faith.

PRACTICE EXAMPLE 10.1: BUILDING
A GIANT PUDSEY BEAR

One of the amazing experiences I had was working alongside the
youth workers in the hospital with a youth group from a mental
health ward. Facilitated by a student on placement, they built a
giant Pudsey bear to celebrate an annual BBC fundraising initiative,
Children in Need, and they had a strong focus on the downward
dimension – how could they raise money to help other children and
young people who had significant needs. They set up in the corridor
near the main entrance and sold lots of things they had made at
youth club. The outwards and inwards dimensions were particularly
significant.

Sally Nash, chaplaincy volunteer

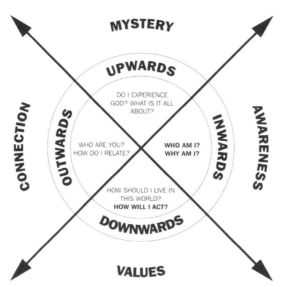

Figure 10.1: Quaker Spiritual Development Model
Source: Lee 2007

Kessler's seven gateways

Kessler identifies seven gateways to spiritual development with young
people: the yearning for deep connection, the longing for silence and
solitude, the search for meaning and purpose, the hunger for joy and
delight, the creative drive, the urge for transcendence, the need for

initiation (2000, p.17). Research suggests (Wilson 2004) that young people find everyday activities spiritual, and while there may be times when we identify one of these gateways as part of our approach, they may often occur in our everyday encounters with children and young people as we build on the skills that we have in communicating with them and have a spiritual moment. Young people mentioned activities such as talking with friends, listening to music and watching the stars as being spiritual, because they contribute to their sense of wellbeing and wholeness, a sense of transcendence and oneness with the world and others (Wilson 2004). Spiritually oriented activities (whether religious or not) have been shown to be of benefit to young people in areas such as helping them feel calmer, focus better, think more clearly and processing bad experiences (Wilson 2002).

Spiritual wellbeing

As spiritual care practitioners, one of our potential aims is to enhance the spiritual wellbeing of those we work with. There are always going to be dimensions of life which impact this, however (drawing on the work of one of the authors in Nash and Pimlott 2010, p.12), we understand spiritual wellbeing to be:

> a sense of satisfaction and contentment with life indicated by an inner peace, self acceptance, the capacity to encounter the transcendent, a sense of connectedness to and engagement with nature, a wider community and the world and a sense of purpose and meaning in and for life including a feeling of empowerment to make a difference.

Although spirituality as the essence of humanity and a key component of our wellbeing has not been central to Western thinking in recent centuries, it is fascinating to note that it is a commonly held worldview preserved in many indigenous people groups where poor wellbeing would primarily be associated with an impoverished spirit. A review of research into wellbeing (Aked *et al.* 2008) suggests that there are five everyday activities that can enhance our wellbeing, which are:

- connect to people
- be physically active
- take notice
- keep learning
- give.

In our hospital context we cannot always do much about the second one but each of the other areas can be built into our spiritual care plans. Our research with young cancer patients particularly demonstrated the importance of the capacity to give to others, which helps with both connectedness and learning. Taking notice is perhaps the area which we can readily do as part of our every day conversations and interactions with children and young people, and we may want to:

- be curious

- catch sight of the beautiful

- remark on the unusual

- notice the changing seasons

- savour the moment

- reflect on our experiences.

(Aked *et al.* 2008)

Spiritual concerns, spiritual distress, spiritual despair

While spiritual wellbeing is what we are working towards, we may well encounter people experiencing spiritual concerns, distress or despair. Hughes and Handzo (2010, p.18) have some useful definitions of these areas using a broad understanding of 'spiritual'. While they are not child specific, they are relevant:

> Spiritual concerns are the potential disruption of one's beliefs, assumptions, or values that occurs when one's valued relationship with one's self, others, ideas, nature, higher power, art, or music is threatened or challenged.

> Spiritual distress is the disruption of one's beliefs, assumptions, or values that occurs when one's valued relationship with one's self, others, ideas, nature, higher power, art, or music is threatened or broken.

> Spiritual despair is the dissolution and/or disintegration of one's source of meaning and hope, leading to one's feeling little to no hope of resolution.

So a child or young person being less engaged with their music, for example, may be an indicator that something is wrong and that there are some spiritual concerns which would benefit from being explored.

In our work in hospital, this is likely, and spiritual distress may be the consequence of a particular diagnosis or experience of treatment. All three of these dimensions can be encountered in the families of sick children and young people as well.

PRACTICE EXAMPLE 10.2: SPIRITUAL
STRUGGLE – PRAYER BOOK

Looking at our prayer books and prayer leaves in chapel gives vivid examples of spiritual struggles:

> I am not a religious person, but I'm asking you to make my little girl better. She has been in pain for 5 months. We have been here now 3 weeks and she seems to get better then something else happens. She has been unbelievably brave and takes everything thrown at her. Our three children are the most precious things in our lives. Please make her better I am begging you.

Facilitating spiritual conversations

Rebecca Nye, a leading expert on child spirituality, has helped us at BCH to develop the skill of having significant spiritual conversations with children and young people. This is what she shared with us around two key concerns: 'I don't know *what* to say to them' and '*How* can these conversations happen then?'

I don't know what to say to them

Don't worry! Spiritual conversation is more about being fully present, attentive and listening rather than saying special things or knowing 'the right questions'. Even though children's language is less developed than an adult's, and they might have a small vocabulary and knowledge of spiritual matters, research shows that children can put spiritual issues and experience into words. Much more than clever spiritual openers and prompts, what children need from us is the sense that we notice, listen and take seriously their many ways of knowing about life, and any meaning they draw from that.

How can these conversations happen then?

BE AWARE OF YOUR OWN SPIRITUAL STATE/MOOD

A genuine conversation is a meeting of two or more people. So, a 'significant spiritual conversation' involves your spirituality as well as the child's. How you are will impact on the quality of the encounter – how much you notice, what seems meaningful or not and much more.

BE AWARE OF YOUR VIEW OF CHILDREN'S SPIRITUALITY

Every meeting with others involves our assumptions about them, try to be aware of what these are for meeting with *this* child. Notice if these are likely to helpfully amplify or unhelpfully attenuate your sensitivity any spirituality they might share.

BE INTENTIONAL ABOUT CREATING A GOOD, WELL-PROTECTED SPACE FOR THE CONVERSATION

Spiritually significant dialogue will dig, it is hoped, quite deep and may perhaps travel into risky or difficult places. So the place it starts from, and finishes in, needs to feel as safe as possible. Consider how the time and space for the meeting can be protected from interruptions – perhaps a sign to other staff/visitors could be used for the duration of the visit. Be prepared to be an advocate for the child if there is an interruption – doing so signals this *is* significant. A spiritual conversation might be thought of as a moment of sanctuary?

If possible, avoid being positioned face to face; sitting at right angles to the child is easier for them. This gives a sense of interpersonal closeness but also necessary personal space directly in front of the child. Spiritual conversation can offer quite a lot of reflection – so it's good to avoid being the main object in the child's view! If they are drawing or doing some other expressive activity, it also gives the main focus to what is directly in front of them, with you more alongside.

BALANCE 'BEING NATURAL' WITH THE SPECIAL DEMANDS OF SPIRITUAL CONVERSATION

Timing and pace may be different. To a large extent, these conversations thrive on being natural, authentic, ordinary chats rather than anything 'weird'! But, they do make different demands on us, especially children. It is not like talking about the weather or what we like to eat. Often spiritual feelings and thoughts have never been put into words before, or coming into consciousness in the present moment. Give extra time for the extra processing and reflection all this needs. Voicing these kinds of thoughts may be a spiritual experience in its own right – not just comments about their spirituality. The usual pace of normal conversation might *not* facilitate things so well.

So, we can help children by slowing down, pausing to 'take things in', speaking a little more quietly, and perhaps encouraging them so that they can 'think' before they say anything (e.g. if doing an activity like choosing a blob or talking about a postcard). By modelling this slower reflective style, you can facilitate the child's use of the same approach. Bear in mind, voicing some spiritual things involves not just *finding* significant things in our experience, but also *making decisions* about whether to tell someone, or not. All that takes more time than ordinary conversations. (Note: Sometimes children might need to test you out with a trial-run comment about something else – for example, a crazy fantasy. If you take that seriously and reflectively, they might feel more able to open up with other things. This might take up all of one conversation/meeting.)

'Wasting time' together is a valuable tool in creating the rapport that may signal it's safe to address spiritual matters. Don't expect spiritual conversations to stay on task for long: sometimes it seems children need to step back from the heat, as if the spiritual temperature gets too hot for them, and change the subject. Respect that. Having significant spiritual conversations is more about quality than quantity.

USE NON-VERBAL COMMUNICATION WHENEVER POSSIBLE

Respect silence. As soon as things are going, a golden rule is to say as little as possible (as well as leaving good pauses before you do say the next thing). All conversations thrive on non-verbal cues, and children are especially sensitive to these. The best support for children's talk, as well as their internal thoughts you might not hear, is to *show* you are interested but give main use of the auditory space to them. Listening with your ears, eyes, gestures, in fact your whole body posture, can support a child to 'carry on' or not. So, rather than say 'tell me about your picture', see if you can try to 'say' that with your face, non-verbally – with a smile, a quizzical look, tracing your finger over the paper thoughtfully, with wonder, implying you sense there's depth there, and so on. Try to see this powerful way of speaking without words as significant spiritual conversation in itself. If the child does not go on to speak about their picture or craft, perhaps that's because words have nothing to add to the meaning they've made here and now, and that in fact words (theirs or ours) could dilute or dissolve that. This has implications for what we might say to the child when ending the encounter. Facilitative work includes communicating that you've 'heard' more than just what the child *said*. For example, 'I'm grateful for the time you spent drawing with me here today,' or 'It was so good to watch you playing/making today, you seemed really into that,' or 'The storytime we had together just now felt very special.'

When a child's response in conversation is silence, be aware this could mean many things. For instance, that they don't *want* to speak about that, that they find it too *hard* to speak about that (perhaps they don't understand), that they don't have anything to say, or that the child recognises this topic demands a response that is deeper than words. A helpful motto for the adult in this instance is the Quaker phrase, 'speak only to improve the silence!' Don't judge your 'success' by how much is said.

INTERPRETING WHEN THINGS *ARE* SAID

With children, and with children's spirituality in particular, the gap between when we hear and the thought they are hoping to convey can be very large! The best approach is to assume the verbalised thought is the tip of an iceberg – that there's unimaginable depth beneath it; even if you can't check that out for certain, it's best to take a generous perspective.

When adults recollect times in childhood when they had spiritual insights and experiences, a common theme is that they felt hardly able to say anything about it at the time and so felt it was weirdly invisible to their parents/teachers, etc., yet felt it was simultaneously intensely vivid to them. For example, a man recalls telling his mum, when he was about 4, 'We're all ants on a giant's tummy you know,' trying to convey a whole process of thinking and insight that had arisen from watching some ants in the garden, thinking about the size of the universe and whether or not there was a caring, creating power that looked out for these ants, and for him. It's probably safe to assume not just an iceberg underneath, but also that children's spirituality can have even more intensity than the spiritual feelings and insights of adults.

It can be hard to be sure you both are using words in the same way. The child's *own* use language and meaning needs to be 'king' to facilitate depth and richness. By checking out what the child means by a particular word, an important message about power is given – in this moment the child's meaning and lived experience refers to matters more than the dictionary definition or correcting their vocabulary!

The *content* is often not such a good clue to knowing if there might be an iceberg below what a child says in conversation with us. Instead, pay attention to the *manner* in which it's said – the energy, the emphasis, things said as statements, things said as questions, things said playfully, and so on.

Develop the habit of noticing the questions a child asks – these are a great sign of where the sources of their energy and curiosity are. Notice *every* question (Where did you get your necklace? Do you know everyone's name? Do you know where I got my teddy from?) – not just ones that seem relevant. What do they suggest about what matters to this child right now? And, since spiritual life is much more about journey and process than arrival and end product, a great way to facilitate spiritual conversation is to really value questioning as a key skill. So, rather than immediately supporting children to find their own answers, perhaps first focus on holding their significant questions 'up to the light' (e.g. repeat it back: 'That's such an interesting question, you've asked a question whole books are written about. I'd like to write that question down to really think about it').

KEEPING THE CONVERSATION GOING

Something to avoid if possible is the sense of spiritual conversation as a one-off. If there has been some opening up, it's unlikely that it all felt 'finished' and complete in one session. There may be afterthoughts, good and bad. It could feel that the person who's heard the child's intimate soul thoughts have been 'taken away', like a physical specimen! That is where leaving something with the child from an activity provides some ongoing continuity with the conversation experience and a container for the child's afterthoughts, either in the hospital or when they go home. Equally, it can be helpful to signal to the child how *you* will hold that conversation, that child, in mind after it stops (e.g. writing the child's name/questions in a special notebook, taking a photo of the child's artwork and explaining about the special place in which you keep these and go on thinking about them).

Summary

- Spiritual literacy involves reflecting on our own spiritual journey.

- There are models that are useful in exploring spirituality and which may inform spiritual care and the development of spiritual care activities.

- Spiritual conversation is an integral part of spiritual care and there are insights which help us do this more effectively.

Conclusion

Sore to soar – lifting spirits

Most of us have heard or used the phrase 'that really lifted my spirit'. This is as close as we have come to explaining what we hope happens within young people when spiritual care is offered. We frequently find that using activities creates space and opportunity for children and young people to voice and share their concerns, hopes, dreams, or anything which is on their mind, and spiritual care practitioners listen, engage with and respond to what emerges. In this book, we have put forward principles, good practice and exercises which will enable effective spiritual care to be offered. All of this is within the framework of ISE, interpretive spiritual encounters, which offer both assessment and intervention as we work towards giving attention to the spiritual dimension of the children and young people in our hospital. We have also found that these approaches work well with adults and we have used many of the activities with family members, but also with staff. Spiritual care is a multidisciplinary responsibility and different disciplines can learn from each other as we seek to provide a child-focused service which enhances spiritual wellbeing. We try to offer an asset-focused approach that builds on what we find in the children and young people, and their families, and which affirms and encourages them as the unique human beings that they are.

Although we have learnt so much about spiritual care with sick children and young people, we recognise that this is only the beginning, and with regard to developing the field of paediatric spiritual care, enhancing spiritual wellbeing and ensuring the highest standards of practice we need to continue to build upon our and others' experience. Our next area of development is to research which of our ISE activities is most suitable for a first contact with someone and to be able to make suggestions as to what further intervention would be helpful as part of a spiritual care plan. We are also committed in the long term to seeking to develop spiritual care standards for paediatric chaplaincy. These are elements of the Centre for Paediatric Spiritual Care, which we have established at BCH, and which includes materials for spiritual care which we publish under the Red Balloon Resources banner. The Centre also offers training courses and participation days where it is possible to come and work alongside us. Our aspirational vision and objectives include the following:

- Spiritual care is integrated into all healthcare staff roles.

- We understand the overlap and synergy of multidisciplinary spiritual care.

- Multidisciplinary paediatric spiritual care standards are developed.

- Increase understanding of the particular spiritual needs according to condition or illness.

- Finding and agreeing a common language to engage with and record spiritual care.

- Research into the benefits of offering spiritual care and how it affects and interacts with physical and psychological needs.

- Developing with children and young people, families and staff further resources that support and facilitate the above.

Spiritual care with sick children and young people begins with creating space and opportunity for conversation, activities and for trust to be built. Being aware of our own spiritual journey and how this impacts our capacity to offer spiritual care and, where necessary, religious care facilitates our effectiveness. Spiritual care is a non-judgmental, accepting, affirming, attentive activity which requires our full presence and the offering of respect and the gaining of ongoing consent. Spiritual care takes place individually or in small groups, at the bedside, in specialist play areas, school, faith rooms or other appropriate places. Offering choice and empowering children helps them develop autonomy in an environment where little may be available. Creativity and a willingness to improvise can be helpful in making the most of an opportunity. What emerges from activities needs to be treated with reverence and respect and young people need to understand what happens with what they have created or entrusted to the spiritual care practitioner. The whole family can engage in spiritual care activities, which they can be adapted to be used by people of all abilities and situations. Spiritual care is a reciprocal activity and as spiritual care practitioners we gain much from the encounters and can be profoundly moved and changed by our engagement with spiritual care. This is a privilege which we never take for granted.

Appendix 1
Spiritual Care Activity Recording Sheet
BCH Chaplaincy Case Study

Name: _____ Age: ____ Gender: ____

Ward:_____ Date: _____

(Recorded) faith: _____ Staff member: _____

Duration of contact: _____

1. Background	How was the child referred to you/how do you know the child? How many times have you seen the child before this encounter? Have you had any interaction with the family? If so, what? Why is the child in hospital? Are there factors affecting the intervention, e.g. learning or physical disabilities, language difficulties, mental health issues?
2. Religious assessment	How did you know there was faith/religion? *(Evidence of faith may include artefacts, dress, conversation)*

3. Spiritual assessment	*(Spirituality may include: attachment/belonging; connectedness/family/relationships/community/friends; purpose; beliefs and rituals; sense of security and identity, sense of hope/hopelessness – what is important to the child's sense of self; feelings – guilt, anger, fear, love, vulnerability, shame, anxieties, hopes; sense of the sacred)* How did you know these were issues? What resources does the child bring to this?
4. Intervention	What did you do? *(Describe the whole sequence of your encounter; at what points and in what ways was your intervention 'intentional'?)* How did it begin? *(Entering, greeting)* What did you do/what happened? *(e.g. activity)* Closure? Why did you choose this intervention?

5. Spiritual care principles	Please tick:
	☐ Building relationship with trusted adult
	☐ Building relationship with God or transcendent other
	☐ Feeling connected and valued
	☐ Feeling listened to and affirmed
	☐ Knowing what/who is important to the child
	☐ Feeling cared for
	☐ Taken seriously; empowered
	☐ Offered a non-medical experience of life
	☐ Building self-esteem; helping children feel good about themselves
	☐ Explore the feelings of the child (worries, hopes, fears, anger, guilt, joys)
	☐ Share fun; play
	☐ Adding to the child's richness of experience
	☐ Sense of purpose and meaning
	☐ Exploring the sacred
	☐ Nurturing rituals and beliefs

6. Assessment of intervention	*(Including feedback from child and/or family)*
	What did you observe during the intervention? What positive or negative body language is important to note?
	Any notable quotations or actions that reflect the effectiveness (or lack of) of the intervention?
	Did the child/this intervention also provide spiritual care for *you*/others? If so, describe this...
7. Moments of grace	When or where was there a moment of 'ordinary grace'? *(This describes instances when a sense of the immediate/ordinary and ultimate/extraordinary coincide somehow. It may be intuited/felt by you rather than explicitly what was said/happened. It may be a clue for what was 'spiritual' in your encounter)*

8. What went well/what could be improved?	What went well/what could be improved?
	What future interventions may be appropriate?
	What other information would have been helpful?
	Are there additional resources or training needed?
9. Key insights	What were the learning outcomes?
	What specific insights are there for that particular child?
	What general insights are there for our practice more widely?
	Are there any actions that should be implemented as a result of this intervention?
	Are there any issues to be discussed at a staff meeting or in supervision?

10. Gaining consent/assent	How did you obtain consent or assent? Video ☐ Photos ☐ Were there any issues with this? If so, how did you overcome them?

Appendix 2
Sample Activity Instructions

Bead Bracelets (children and young person instructions)
Materials: various beads, thread to string beads on, scissors, activity sheet.

Make a bracelet for your spiritual care
Make a bracelet for the things you need, want or feel while you are sick or in hospital.

> Green = peace
>
> Red = that I matter
>
> White = hope for the future
>
> Pink = strength
>
> Purple = faith in God
>
> Brown = honesty
>
> Blue = happiness
>
> Orange = to be able to help others
>
> Yellow = I belong
>
> Heart-shaped = I am loved/wanted

MY COLOURS, MY MEANINGS (WHAT THEY MEAN TO ME)
Why have you put those particular colours on your bracelet? Think about what you already have, what you are able to offer to others and how you might be able to have what you would like. Is there anything that you would like to pray about: to give thanks to God for or ask God to help you with?

Make a bracelet for your Islamic spiritual care
Make a bracelet for the things you need to have, want or feel while you are sick or in hospital.

> Silver = patience; have *sabr*
>
> Red = that I matter

Pink = strength

White = hope for the future

Black/purple = faith in God

Brown = honesty

Orange = to be able to help others

Green = happiness

Blue = peace

Yellow = to be noticed

Gold = I belong/I am wanted

Heart-shaped = I am loved

MY COLOURS, MY MEANINGS (WHAT THEY MEAN TO ME)

Why have you put those particular colours on your bracelet? Think about what you already have, what you are able to offer to others and how you might be able to have what you would like. Is there anything that you would like to pray about: to give thanks to Allah (show *shukr*) or ask Allah to help you with?

Beads in a mental health context

Make a bracelet for the things you need, want or feel in hospital.

LARGE BEADS – WHAT I WANT/MY FUTURE

Dark green = peace

Red = to feel that I matter

Pink = strength to get help

Purple = faith in God

Brown = I want to be honest

Heart shaped = to feel I am loved/wanted

Peach = to feel appreciated

Orange = to be able to help others

Yellow = to feel I belong somewhere

Blue = happiness in all I do

Light green = to feel safe

White = hope for the future

SMALL BEADS – WHAT I FEEL/MY PRESENT (NOW)

Green = scared/frightened

Red = worried about something

White = I need help with something, but don't know how to ask

Pink = feel unwell/poorly

Blue = confused about something

Purple = someone hurts me/bullies me

Black = I don't want to be here anymore. I wish I was dead

Clear bead = worried about money

Sparkly bead = I want to hurt/cut myself

Tubular bead = upset/worried about school

Coloured-star bead = nervous about something

Spotty bead = feelings about food

Orange = drugs/alcohol

Silver star = feel lonely/isolated

Brown = sex/boys/girls

Yellow = angry

Love = someone makes me feel special

Person bead = problems at home (family)

MY COLOURS, MY MEANINGS (WHAT THEY MEAN TO ME)

Why have you put those particular colours on your bracelet? Think about what you already have, what you are able to offer to others and how you might be able to have what you would like.

Blob Tree Activity (team instructions)

Materials: clay, playdough, plasticine or similar material to make the blobs, material to make leaves, if required, some blob pictures to begin with and a skeleton tree.

Principles

- Let the children and young people direct the play and follow their lead.

- Let the children interpret the meaning – you can ask questions about the blob they have designed and where they place the blob on the tree – avoid assuming meaning – just ask!

- Let them make the expression on the face (choose colour, etc.) – this can be very revealing; again, avoid suggestions.

- There are no real rules about the tree – young people will have their own design ideas and this will be part of the self-exploration.

- Participate yourself. Design your own self-portrait (as long as you are not too absorbed!). This also shows that you are willing to share something of who you are. You will also see how it feels to do what you are asking the children and young people to do.

Beginning

Think about how you will start the session. Create a safe space:

- Simple introduction to each other; all together in a circle.

- Introduce the activity simply – tell them what will happen with their figure at the end.

What will you do?

- Start with choosing one blob picture – find yourself in one of the pictures too!

- This will warm the children up to the activity.

- Gently introduce the idea of identifying with the blobs.

- Ask questions about their picture and their choice.

Move on to making our own blobs (and Blob Tree is part of the activity) and invite the young people to place their blob(s) wherever they want to, encouraging them to explain their blob and where they have placed it.

Closure

Think about how you are going to round off the session.

- Remember that you may have opened up some difficult and sensitive feelings.

- Take time to praise and enjoy what has been created.

- Explain where the tree is being stored or displayed.

- Consider taking photographs of the children and young people with their blob, both on and off the tree.

Elephant in the Room (team instructions)

Materials: elephants, pens, paint, glue, decopatch paper, etc., shoe boxes to create room.

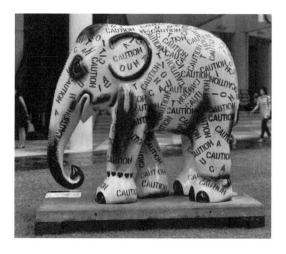

The project is based on the idea that an elephant in a room would be impossible to overlook; thus, people in the room who pretend the elephant is not there have chosen to avoid dealing with the looming big issue. Invite the children/young people to read the poem quietly to themselves or read it aloud – whichever they feel more comfortable with. They are then invited to decorate an elephant using various mediums, pens, decopatch, paint, etc. They can use any medium they like to express the metaphorical elephant in the room. The representation can be either literal on the elephant or they can use colours, pictures and so on to decorate it. An alternative suggestion, if they would not like to use an elephant, is to design an elephant footprint which can be displayed to represent their elephant. All the elephants and footprints with permission will be displayed.

Things to be aware of
Children/young people/parents may not want to address the elephant in the room.

Issues that may arise

I don't feel safe	Why me?
I feel lonely	I'm bored
My friend died	Will I be home for my birthday?
When will I get home?	Why am I sick?
My school friends might forget me	Get some perspective, don't sweat the small stuff!
I might not get better	I don't feel safe/at night
Why me?	Do I matter?
Is this my fault?	

Follow up
Staff participating in this project need to have the capacity to do follow-up visits as required. The emotions/issues which may come to the surface may need further visits and reflection time. Young people may need help to process these feelings and what is being said, and the family will need support in discussing issues with their children, which they were previously happy to leave as an 'elephant'.

Referral forward
If you feel the issues you have dealt with are complex and out of your skills remit please use a referral form for the CAMHS service.

Child protection concerns
Due to the sensitive nature of the topics which may occur during discussions, all staff facilitating this event need to have completed child protection training and read the Childline report, *Saying the Unsayable* (Childline 2012) for an up-to-date summary of issues and concerns children and young people are currently facing.

Writing in multidisciplinary team (MDT) notes

This project sits between different specialities – some of which write in MDT notes and some which do not. Whilst there are valid arguments for practices on both sides linked to the professions they work for, within this project all professions need to explain to those involved that disclosures made may need to be taken further, written in the MDT notes and discussed with their named nurse/doctor. This then gives the child/young person a choice whether to reveal certain information or not.

Examen Doll: Looking back on my day (team instructions)

Materials: stick figure, pens, activity sheet. These wooden stick people are about the length of a usual lolly stick and the figure is around 4cm wide. One source of these is www.hobbycraft.co.uk/hobbycraft-create-and-play-wooden-people/574562-1000.

Invite a child or young person to prepare a wooden figure (lolly-stick style, male or female).

1. Draw and colour in the hair, eyes, mouth and nose, and any clothing and shoes they would like, using gel pens or special ink pens provided.

2. On one side, make a happy face. On the other side, make a sad face.

3. When was I happiest today? (Write this question on the happy face side of your stick.)

4. When was I saddest today? (Write this question on the sad face side of your stick.)

There are other ways to ask the same questions; choose the version most appropriate:

For what moment today am I most grateful? What was today's high point?

For what moment today am I least grateful? What was today's low point?

When did I give and receive the most love today?

When did I give and receive the least love today?

Take a few minutes to demonstrate the exercise:

1. Become quiet together (do whatever helps you to relax: take a few deep breaths, imagine your body filled with light; breathe in love).

2. Think about the events of the day. Notice when you felt most happy and when you felt most sad.

3. Share with your parent or carer your answers, using your doll to remind you of the times when you felt happiest/saddest.

4. Maybe your parent would also like to think about their day, and share their thoughts.

5. If you say prayers, you could thank God for the happy moments, and ask God to help you with anything that is difficult.

You may also have time to help the child to design a bag for keeping their doll in, using fabric pens and small bags.

Do remember

-   Some children may have very difficult material to share from their day. Don't be alarmed! Receive their story, and if you need to share anything with another member of staff, explain to the child first that you are going to do this in order to support them better.

-   Even on the most difficult days, there is usually some moment of happiness. Remembering these can help engender hope and resilience for children and young people.

Examen Doll: Looking back on my day (child and young person instructions)

First of all, choose a wooden doll, male or female. Draw and colour in the hair, eyes, mouth and nose, and any clothing and shoes you would like. Make it special, just like you! On one side, make a happy face. On the other side, make a sad face. Use these two sides to help you think about two questions:

When was I happiest today? (Write this question on the happy face side of your stick.)

When was I saddest? (Write this question on the sad face side of your stick.)

There are other ways to ask the same question:

> What was today's high point? What was today's low point?
>
> When did I give and receive the most love today?
>
> When did I give and receive the least love today?

Doing the exercise

1. Take a moment to become quiet and still.

2. Play back the events of the day in your mind. Notice when you felt happy and when you felt sad.

3. When was the happiest moment? When was the saddest?

4. Share your answers with your parent or carer. Maybe your parents would like to think about their day and tell you their thoughts.

5. If you say prayers, you could thank God for the happy moments, and ask God to help you with anything that is difficult.

You might like to make a special bag to keep your doll in for another day.

Hope Blanket (family instructions)

Would you like to design a patch for our Hope Blanket? Make your own unique design!

The theme of the blanket is: What gives your family hope? What are you hoping or dreaming for at this time? Can you think of one or several things to draw or design on your fabric patch? You can stick on pictures from magazines or the internet, glue on bits of fabric, paper, sequins or other decorative things, or even try your hand at sewing!

Please note: the patches will be collected together and woven into a Hope Blanket. This will be displayed in the hospital chapel. You can have both a photo of your patch and of the completed blanket if you would like. Just ask the leader.

Sensory Boxes (team instructions)

Materials: blank or patterned boxes, things to decorate box with: stickers, fake jewels, etc., selection of things to put in the boxes relating to the five senses.

1. Invite your child to prepare a sensory box.

2. Dress up and decorate the box – make it their own – a unique reflection of the unique person that they are.

3. Fill the box with items that bring comfort and fun – something the children or young people can look at and enjoy, especially if they are having a low moment, or feel bored. They can turn to their box of favourite things.

Think about the five senses

TASTE
Sweets; hot chocolate mix; special treats or drinks; flavoured lip balm; box of special cereal; chewing gum.

TOUCH
Soft toy; scarf; pretty material; stress ball; smooth rubbing stone; hand lotion; beads; bracelet.

HEARING
Rustling paper; homemade paper; CD with favourite music; small instrument, e.g. shaker, harmonica.

SMELL
Essential oil on cotton wool; smelly candle; incense stick; spices in a jar, e.g. cinnamon; body lotion; lip balm.

SIGHT
Postcard from a favourite place; photo of family, pet, friends; special birthday card; nature scene; favourite colour; drawing/collage of favourite things; pretty material; scarf.

Questions to ask
What makes you feel better? What makes you giggle? What is your favourite colour? What is your favourite music? What does your favourite place look like?

Spiritual Care Bandage (team instructions)
Materials: bandages – tube ones can be used to make bracelets, fabric pens.

Invite the children or young people to write on the bandage what they need or would like to feel while they are in hospital. They can then decorate the bandage with other materials. Their bandage bracelet can then be worn as a positive reminder of what they hope will happen or what they will experience. It may also act as a prompt for them to consider how these things could occur or to ask for help with them. A further idea is that they make copies of their spiritual care bandage to send home for their friends. The importance of connection and connectivity emerges in recent research and this will help us to interact with children and young people in relation to this potential spiritual need.

If prompts are needed, these are some of the things that may be written on the bandages:

- strength
- cared for
- happy
- peace
- to go home
- family with me
- hope
- loved
- patience
- trust in God
- not be on my own
- able to help others
- make new friends
- listened to
- get better
- privacy
- be less bored
- see more friends

- time and space for myself

- to be able to be me

- not forgotten/remembered at home

- get used to how I am now

What other words might they want to write?

Prompts for discussing the bandage

Why have you put those particular words on your bandage? Think about what you already have, and then what you would like to have. Perhaps write what they have and feel already on one side and what they want to feel like on the other. How might they be able to feel or have more of what they would like? What could they/others do?

Imagery: bind up, strap up.

Suggestion: Place some paper under the bandage because of seepage.

Copy some to send home to school friends

Perhaps they would like to send a copy of their own bandage, or something like it, home for their friends to wear. Children could ask their friends to wear it to remember or pray for what the child wants to feel like. This will mean their friends are always thinking of them even when they do not see the child. The bandages are washable.

Information for home

The bandages were all new and sealed before the child writes on them and are washable. We suggest they are worn by only one person to help with hygiene issues. Wearing them will help the child or young person who created them feel that they are not forgotten. It can be an act of solidarity with them.

Principles, Practice Examples and Activities Grid

Activities	Practice examples
Principle 1: Participation, empowerment and autonomy are core underpinning values of spiritual care	
3.1 Dream jar	4.1 Janine's story
4.3 Being a journalist	4.6 Praying with Jack
5.3 Islamic bead bracelets	5.5 Dani's faces
5.4 Sensory box	7.7 Maddy's trip to hospital
	9.2 To share or not to share?
	9.3 Empowering Younas
Principle 2: We need to create spaces for spiritual care to occur (most of our activities and examples reflect this)	
5.1 Singing and dancing – fun as spiritual care	3.2 Facilitating spiritual wellbeing
5.4 Sensory box	5.2 Working with a sibling
5.6 Easter chicks	7.4 In the bereavement suite
6.5 Safe space	7.11 Spiritual care for bereaved families
7.2 Simple questionnaires	8.1 Working with Kara
8.1 Relaxation and visualisation exercises	8.5 Singing with newborns
	9.4 Activities that promote wellbeing and self-care
	9.5 Staff support
	10.2 Spiritual struggle – prayer book
Principle 3: Spiritual care occurs within the context of relationship	
All of our activities and examples reflect this	3.1 Another box for Ria
	4.2 Lizzie's beads – what's important in life
	5.4 Lauren's candle holder
	6.4 Ben's lantern
	7.3 Mirium's beads
	9.1 Lilly's operation
	9.2 To share or not to share?

Principle 4: Spiritual care happens in the context of family and often with family present

5.5	Spiritual care blankets	4.3	Heaven backwards
6.1	Stone painting	4.4	Marigold's family
6.6	Decorating a tea light holder	6.2	Dilan's story (part 1)
6.7	Making a jigsaw	7.1	Working with Mia
7.1	Hope blanket	7.2	Sioned and her dad
7.3	Family caring tree	7.4	In the bereavement suite
7.4	Paper flowers	7.5	Sara's Dream Space
8.8	Gold hearts	7.9	Multidisciplinary working
		7.10	Watching Sam and his special book
		7.11	Spiritual care for bereaved families
		7.12	Ali's cricket Dream Space
		8.9	Annie and the Good Shepherd

Principle 5: We need to connect and build on existing spirituality and, if appropriate, faith

4.2	God's daisy	3.1	Another box for Ria
5.6	Easter chicks	4.4	Marigold's family
8.1	Relaxation and visualisation exercises	4.6	Praying with Jack
8.2	Multisensory quiet time	5.3	Art activities with Sonam
8.3	Easter garden	5.4	Lauren's candle holder
8.4	Imagining God	6.8	Nathaniel's Easter story bracelet
8.5	Prayer stones	7.1	Working with Mia
8.6	Religious bracelets	7.2	Sioned and her dad
8.7	Labyrinth postcard	7.9	Multidisciplinary working
9.1	The window	8.2	Dilan's story (part 2) – religious care
9.2	Mandalas	8.3	Josefina's prayer
10.1	Exploring our own spiritual journey	8.6	Blessing Kate
		8.10	Briar Tinkerbell and a light for Nanny
		8.11	Josefina's story

Principle 6: Developmental and learning context is important to understand in choosing activities, resources and language	
4.4 Teddy goes to hospital 5.7 Dream Space 8.2 Multisensory quiet time	4.2 Lizzie's beads – what's important in life 5.5 Dani's faces 6.5 Working with Holly 7.6 Becky's sensory box 7.8 Sian's painting 7.10 Watching Sam and his special book 8.5 Singing with newborns 8.6 Blessing Kate 8.7 Singing with Wilf 8.8 Soothing Marcus

Principle 7: Metaphor can be a significant tool for spiritual care	
5.7 Dream Space 6.1 Stone painting 6.2 Chess as a metaphor for dying 6.4 Elephant in the Room 8.3 Easter garden 8.5 Prayer stones 9.4 Vomit bowl and locker 9.5 Pelican card 9.6 What's the weather like today?	6.3 We are diamonds 6.6 Paula going home

Principle 8: Spiritual care occurs within and by a community and can offer windows of normalisation	
4.3 Being a journalist 6.6 Decorating a tea light holder 6.7 Making a jigsaw 6.8 3D Blob tree 6.9 My favourite day 7.2 Simple questionnaires 7.4 Paper flowers	3.2 Facilitating spiritual wellbeing 5.1 Omar's snowball fight 5.3 Art activities with Sonam 8.4 Singing medicine 8.7 Singing with Wilf 10.1 Building a giant Pudsey bear

Principle 9: Meaning making helps children and young people articulate, identify and understand their spiritual needs

3.1	Dream jar	1.1	Ria's box
4.1	What is important to you?	4.2	Lizzie's beads
4.4	Teddy goes to hospital	5.2	Working with a sibling
5.3	Islamic bead bracelets	6.1	Peter and Diana's pictures
5.4	Sensory box	6.2	Dilan's story (part 1)
5.6	Easter chicks	6.5	Working with Holly
5.7	Dream Space	6.6	Paula going home
6.3	Blob pictures	6.7	Saying goodbye to Jessica
6.5	Safe space	7.5	Sara's Dream Space (part 2) – religious care
6.8	3D blob tree	8.2	Dilan's story
7.1	Hope blanket	8.9	Annie and the Good Shepherd
8.4	Imagining God	8.10	Briar Tinkerbell and a light for Nanny
8.7	Labyrinth postcard	8.11	Josefina's story
9.2	Mandalas		
9.4	Vomit bowl and locker		
9.6	What's the weather like today?		
10.1	Exploring our own spiritual journey		

Principle 10: Identity may have a heightened significance in sickness

4.2	God's daisy	4.1	Janine's story
9.3	Metaphorical portraits	4.3	Heaven backwards
		4.7	Working with Zach
		6.1	Peter and Diana's pictures
		6.3	We are diamonds
		8.11	Josefina's story

Principle 11: Concrete and visible expressions and reminders of spiritual care are important

5.2	Examen doll	3.1	Another box for Ria
5.3	Islamic bead bracelets	5.4	Lauren's candle holder
5.4	Sensory box	6.4	Ben's lantern
5.5	Spiritual care blankets	6.7	Saying goodbye to Jessica
6.8	3D blob tree	6.8	Nathaniel's Easter story bracelet
7.3	Family caring tree	7.3	Mirium's beads
8.6	Religious bracelets	7.6	Becky's sensory box
8.8	Gold hearts	7.8	Sian's painting
		10.1	Building a giant Pudsey bear

Principle 12: Offering 'episodes of spiritual care' reflects the often integrated nature of assessment and intervention and the element of reciprocity	
5.2 Examen doll	1.1 Ria's box
5.3 Islamic bead bracelets	3.1 Another box for Ria
5.7 Dream Space	5.3 Art activities with Sonam
6.3 Blob pictures	6.1 Peter and Diana's pictures
6.4 Elephant in the Room	6.2 Dilan's story (part 1)
7.3 Family caring tree	7.5 Sara's Dream Space
9.3 Metaphorical portraits	7.12 Ali's cricket Dream Space

Bibliography

Adams, K., Hyde, B. and Woolley, R. (2008) *The Spiritual Dimension of Childhood.* London: Jessica Kingsley Publishers.

Aked, J., Marks, N., Cordon, C. and Thompson, S. (2008) *Five Ways to Well-Being: The Evidence.* London: NEF and the Foresight Commission.

Appleton, L. and Flynn, M. (2014) 'Searching for the new normal: Exploring the role of language and metaphors in becoming a cancer survivor.' *European Journal of Oncology Nursing 18*, 4, 378–384.

Atkinson, T. and Claxton, G. (2000) *The Intuitive Practitioner.* Milton Keynes: Open University Press.

Barritt, P. (2005) *Humanity in Healthcare: The Heart and Soul of Medicine.* Abingdon: Radcliffe.

Beech, V. and the Paediatric Chaplaincy Network (2011) Held in Hope series: *Maya Goes to Hospital; Sam and his Special Book; Josh Stays in Hospital; Jesus Still Loves Joe.* Birmingham: Christian Education.

Bradford, J. (1995) *Caring for the Whole Child: A Holistic Approach to Spirituality.* London: Children's Society.

Bull, A. and Gillies, M. (2007) 'Spiritual needs of children with complex healthcare needs in hospital.' *Paediatric Nursing 19*, 9, 34–38.

Bull, A.W. (2013) 'The Insights Gained from a Portfolio of Spiritual Assessment Tools Used with Hospitalised School-aged Children to Facilitate the Delivery of Spiritual Care Offered by the Healthcare Chaplain.' Unpublished PhD thesis, University of Glasgow.

Campbell, A. (2006) 'Spiritual care for sick children of five world faiths.' *Nursing Children and Young People 18*, 10, 22–25.

Carson, C. and WGRG (1998) 'The Peace of the Earth.' Chicago, IL: GIA Publications.

Carson, M.L.S. (2008) *The Pastoral Care of People with Mental Health Problems.* London: SPCK.

Childline (2012) *Saying the Unsayable.* London: Childline. Available at http://cdn.basw.co.uk/upload/basw_15340-3.pdf, accessed 2 April 2015.

Children's Hospital: The Chaplains (2014) Executive Producer: Julian Mercer. Salford: BBC2, 26 October–30 November 2014.

Children's Society (2014) 'Six Priorities for Children's Well-Being.' Available at www.childrenssociety.org.uk/what-we-do/resources-and-publications/ publications-library/good-childhood-report-2014, accessed on 10 February 2015.

Chislett, V. and Chapman, A. (2005–2012) 'VAK Learning Styles Self-Test.' Available at www.businessballs.com/vaklearningstylestest.htm, accessed on 10 February 2015.

Clarke, J. (2009) 'A critical view of how nursing has defined spirituality.' *Journal of Clinical Nursing 18*, 12, 1666–1673.

Csinos, D.M. and Bellous, J.E. (2009) 'Spiritual styles: Creating an environment to nurture spiritual wholeness.' *International Journal of Children's Spirituality 14*, 3, 213–224.

Darby, K., Nash, P. and Nash, S. (2014a) 'Understanding and responding to spiritual and religious needs of young people with cancer.' *Cancer Nursing Practice 13*, 2, 32–37.

Darby, K., Nash, P. and Nash, S. (2014b) 'Parents' spiritual and religious needs in young oncology.' *Cancer Nursing Practice 13*, 4, 16–22.

Darley, S. and Heath, W. (2008) *Expressive Arts Activity Book*. London: Jessica Kingsley Publishers.

Eaude, T. (2009) 'Happiness, emotional well-being and mental health: What has children's spirituality to offer?' *International Journal of Children's Spirituality 14*, 3, 185–196.

Erickson, D.V. (2008) 'Spirituality, loss and recovery in children with disabilities.' *International Journal of Children's Spirituality 13*, 3, 287–296.

Erikson, E.H. (1995) *Childhood and Society*. London: Vintage.

Feudtner, C., Haney, J. and Dimmers, M.A. (2003) 'Spiritual care needs of hospitalized children and their families: A national survey of pastoral care providers' perceptions.' *Pediatrics 111*, 1, 67–72.

Fisher J. (2011) 'The four domains model: Connecting spirituality, health and well-being.' *Religions 2*, 1, 17–28.

Gardner, H. (1983) *Frames of Mind: The Theory of Multiple Intelligences*. New York, NY: Basic Books.

Griffith, J.L. (2012) 'Psychiatry and Mental Health Treatment.' In M. Cobb, C. Puchalski and B. Rumbold (eds) *Oxford Textbook of Spirituality in Healthcare*. Oxford: University Press.

Grossoehme, D.H. (1996) 'Prayer reveals belief: Images of God from hospital prayers.' *Journal of Pastoral Care 50*, 1, 33–39.

Grossoehme, D.H. (1999) *The Pastoral Care of Children*. New York, NY: Haworth Pastoral Press.

Grossoehme, D.H. (2008a) 'Development of a spiritual screening tool for children and adolescents.' *The Journal of Pastoral Care & Counseling 62*, 1–2, 71–85.

Grossoehme, D.H., Cotton, S. and Leonard, A. (2007a) 'Spiritual and religious experiences of adolescent psychiatric inpatients versus healthy peers.' *The Journal of Pastoral Care & Counseling 61*, 3, 197–204.

Grossoehme, D.H., Szczesniak, R., McPhail, G.L. and Seid, M. (2013) Is adolescents' religious coping with cystic fibrosis associated with the rate of decline in pulmonary function? A preliminary study.' *Journal of Health Care Chaplaincy 19*, 1, 33–42.

Grossoehme, D.H., VanDyke, R. and Seid, M. (2008b) 'Spirituality's role in chronic disease self-management: Sanctification of the body in families dealing with cystic fibrosis.' *Journal of Health Care Chaplaincy 15*, 2, 149–158.

Hart, D. and Schneider, D. (1997) 'Spiritual care for children with cancer.' *Seminars in Oncology Nursing 13*, 4, 263–270.

Hay, D. and Nye, R. (2006) *The Spirit of the Child* (rev. edn). London: Jessica Kingsley Publishers.

Holloway, M. (2006) 'Spiritual need and the core business of social work.' *British Journal of Social Work 37*, 2, 265–280.

Hughes, B. and Handzo, G. (2010) *Spiritual Care Handbook on PTSD/TBI.* Washington, DC: Department of the Navy, Department of Defense, U.S. Government.

Hussain, Z. (2013) *We Will Meet Again in Jannah.* London: Ta-Ha Publishing.

Hyde, B. (2008) *Children and Spirituality.* London: Jessica Kingsley Publishers.

Jacober, A. (2014) 'Adolescent Identity Development.' In S. Nash and J. Whitehead (eds) *Christian Youth Work in Theory and Practice.* London: SCM.

Jason. L.A. (1997) *Community Building.* Westport, CT: Praeger.

Johns, C. (2004) *Becoming a Reflective Practitioner* (2nd edn). Oxford: Blackwell.

Kabat-Zinn, J. (1990) *Full Catastrophe Living Using the Wisdom of Your Body and Mind to Face Stress, Pain, and Illness.* (15th anniversary edn). New York, NY: Bantam Dell.

Kendrick, G. (1988) 'Peace to You.' Tunbridge Wells: Make Way Music.

Kessler, R. (2000) *The Soul of Education.* Alexandria, VA: Association for Supervision and Curriculum Development.

Kettering, T. (undated) 'The Elephant in the Room.' Available at www.irisremembers.com/poemsandstories/viewPoem.cfm?poemID=63, accessed on 10 May 2015.

Lakoff, G. and Johnson, M. (1980) *Metaphors We Live By.* Chicago, IL: University of Chicago Press.

Lee, J. (2007) *Spiritual Development* (2nd edn). London: Quaker Life. Available at www.quaker.org.uk/working-with-12-to-18-years, accessed on 9 May 2015.

Lennon, J. (1980) 'Beautiful Boy (Darling Boy).' On Lennon, J. and Ono, Y. *Double Fantasy* album. Geffen Records.

Liebmann, M. (2004) *Art Therapy for Groups* (2nd edn). Hove: Brunner-Routledge.

Lloyd Webber, A. and Rice, T. (1969) *Joseph and the Amazing Technicolor Dreamcoat.* Decca Records.

McSherry, W. and Cash, K. (2004) 'The language of spirituality: An emerging taxonomy.' *International Journal of Nursing Studies 41*, 2, 151–161.

McSherry, W. and Ross, L. (2010) *Spiritual Assessment in Healthcare Practice.* Keswick: M&K.

Malchiodi, C.A. (1998) *The Art Therapy Sourcebook.* Lincolnwood, IL: Lowell House.

Narayanasamy, A. (2010) 'Recognising Spiritual Needs.' In McSherry, W. and Ross, L. (eds) *Spiritual Assessment in Healthcare Practice.* Keswick: M&K.

Nash, P. (2011) *Supporting Dying Children and their Families.* London: SPCK.

Nash, P., Darby, K. and Nash, S. (2013) 'The spiritual care of sick children: Reflections from a participation project.' *International Journal of Children's Spirituality 18*, 2, 148–161.

Nash, P., Nash, S. and Frith, C. (2011) 'Perspectives on Spirituality and Sick Children and Young People in a Multicultural Paediatric Hospital Context – Identifying and Responding to Spiritual Needs.' Available at www.inter-disciplinary.net/wp-content/uploads/2011/02/nashspaper.pdf, accessed on 10 February 2015.

Nash, P., Parkes, M. and Hussain, Z. (2015) *Multifaith Care for Sick and Dying Children and their Families.* London: Jessica Kingsley Publishers.

Nash, S. (2011) 'Regenerative practice.' *Reflective Practice 12*, 3, 427–438.

Nash, S. (2014) 'Being a Reflective Practitioner and Lifelong Learner: Pursuing Wisdom and Fruitfulness.' In S. Nash and J. Whitehead (eds) *Christian Youth Work in Theory and Practice: A Handbook.* Norwich: SCM Press.

Nash, S. and Pimlott, N. (2010) *Well-being and Spirituality.* Cambridge: Grove.

NHS Education for Scotland (2009) *Spiritual Care Matters: An Introductory Resource for all NHS Scotland staff.* Edinburgh: NES.

O'Connell, D. (2013) *Working with Children and Young People: Good Practice Guidelines for Healthcare Chaplains.* Birmingham: Red Balloon Resources and Paediatric Chaplaincy Network.

Palmer, P.J. (1999) *Let Your Life Speak.* San Francisco, CA: Jossey Bass.

Pattison, S. (2007) *The Challenge of Practical Theology: Selected Essays.* London: Jessica Kingsley Publishers.

Petrie, P. (2011) *Communication Skills for Working with Children and Young People.* London: Jessica Kingsley Publishers.

Pridmore, P. and Pridmore, J.J. (2004) 'Promoting the spiritual development of sick children.' *International Journal of Children's Spirituality 9*, 1, 21–38.

Puchalski, C. and Ferrell, B. (2010) *Making Health Care Whole.* West Conshohocken, PA: Templeton Press.

Robinson, S., Kendrick, K. and Brown, A. (2003) *Spirituality and the Practice of Healthcare.* London: Palgrave Macmillan.

Rogers, C. (1961) *On Becoming a Person.* Constable: London.

Royal College of Nursing (2011) *Spirituality in Nursing Care: A Pocket Guide.* London: Royal College of Nursing. Available at www.rcn.org.uk/__data/assets/pdf_file/0008/372995/003887.pdf, accessed on 10 February 2015.

Scott, P.M. (2013) *My Hospital Prayer and Activities Book.* Chawton: Redemptorist Publications.

Sunderland, M. and Engleheart, P. (1993) *Draw On Your Emotions.* Bicester: Speechmark.

UK Board of Healthcare Chaplaincy (2014) *Spiritual and Religious Care Capabilities and Competences for Chaplaincy Support 2014.* Cambridge: UKBHC. Available at www.ukbhc.org.uk/sites/default/files/ukbhc_spiritual_and_religious_capabilities_and_competences_for_chaplaincy_support_2014.pdf, accessed on 2 April 2015.

Whaley, B.B. (1994) 'Food is to me as gas is to cars? Using figurative language to explain illness to children.' *Health Communication 6*, 3, 193–204.

Williams, M. and Penman, D. (2011) *Mindfulness: A Practical Guide to Finding Peace in a Frantic World.* London: Piatkus.

Wilson, M. (2002) *Practice Unbound.* Boxboro, MA: New England Network for Child, Youth and Family Services.

Wilson, M. (2004) *A Part of You So Deep.* Burlington, VT: New England Network for Child, Youth and Family Services.

Wilson, M. (2005) *Adolescent Heart and Soul.* Burlington. VT: New England Network for Child, Youth and Family Services.

Wilson, P. and Long, I. (2009) *The Big Book of Blobs.* Bicester: Speechmark.

Wolfe, M. (2001) 'Conversation.' In L.D. Richardson and M. Wolfe (eds) *Principles and Practices of Informal Education.* Abingdon: RoutledgeFalmer.

About the Authors

Rev. Paul Nash has worked at Birmingham Children's Hospital since 2002, and has been Chaplaincy Team Leader (Senior Chaplain) since 2004. He is the director of Red Balloon Resources, for paediatric daily, palliative end-of-life and bereavement care for children, families and staff, and the co-founder and co-convenor of the Paediatric Chaplaincy Network for Great Britain and Ireland. He is the academic lead on children's and young people's chaplaincy modules in a partnership with Staffordshire University. His current research involves developing distinctive standards, competencies and best practice for paediatric chaplaincy. Paul lives in Birmingham, UK.

Rev. Kathryn Darby has been a Chaplain at Birmingham Children's Hospital since 2006, is an ordained Methodist Minister and a trained counsellor. She has published research on the spiritual needs of children with cancer and is currently engaged in further research in developing tools for spiritual care with children who are sick. She takes a particular interest in self-care and building resilience for caring professions and runs retreats, mindfulness sessions and projects, including a choir, as part of offering support. She is involved in Spiritual Direction and the Retreat movement. Kathryn lives in Birmingham, UK.

Rev. Dr Sally Nash is an experienced researcher, author and educator. She is Director of the Midlands Institute for Children Youth and Mission and has published in the field of spirituality, spiritual and religious needs of sick children, work with young people, and reflective practice. She is the academic lead for the Birmingham Children's Hospital chaplaincy team on research, designs spiritual care resources and has also been involved as a volunteer in youth work with young people with mental health problems at the hospital. Sally lives in Birmingham, UK

Subject Index

Author Index